The
CARBOSIS
(aka type 2 diabetes)
Owner's Manual and Pocket Guide

Daryl Wein

ISBN: 1491255781
ISBN-13: 978-1491255780
Library of Congress Control Number: 2013914069
CreateSpace Independent Publishing Platform, North Charleston, SC

This Manual is dedicated to all of the "sugar-challenged" patients who have heeded my advice over the years and live relatively healthy lives as a result.

Contents

Acknowledgements

I am deeply grateful to Jan and Richard Moorehouse for their editorial and software assistance. Though I have no trouble planting an airplane on the correct part of a runway I could rarely plant a comma in the right part of a sentence.

Also much appreciation to my new friend, Atra Givarkes, a previously undiscovered young artist with amazing talent. Her thoughtful creation of the image I call "Blanche" will undoubtedly help many "sugar-challenged" people live longer and healthier lives.

Preface

Of all things divinely created, the human body is universally recognized as the most complex. It is a machine of unequalled intricacy. It is remarkably adaptable to change. A hundred years ago machines were compared to the finest of Swiss watches as the gold standard for complexity. Today the most massive of supercomputers pales in comparison with the human brain alone. None can truly think, or reason, or imagine a new song, painting or invention.

Ironically, our advanced intellect has allowed us to devise ways to harm or even destroy ourselves. Many of our destructive concoctions have been intentional, such as weapons for military use. But others have arrived over time through none but the loftiest of intentions. DDT, for example, was a huge boon to agriculture, but far more energy has been expended trying to eradicate this scourge than to develop it in the first place.

Our noble attempts to provide each other delectable treats with long shelf lives has led to the unlimited availability of processed sugar, high-fructose corn syrup, white/bleached flour and polished white rice. Add breakfast cereals, canned fruit juices and year-round fruit and we're faced with a massive overabundance of easily digestible carbohydrate. While some individuals can adapt to safely process these edible bombs, many cannot. The common disease discussed in this manual is just one of several, and perhaps many, disorders directly caused or exacerbated by this overabundance. Fortunately, healthier food choices are still widely available for the many who are genetically predisposed to blood sugar problems or obesity.

This Owner's Manual is provided to help guide the maintenance of the "sugar-challenged" human machine.

Introduction

One of the worst days of my life was sometime in 1998 when I was training to become a Physician Assistant. I was about halfway through school and hadn't reached the point where we studied endocrinology which is the part of medical science that includes diabetes. I had noticed recently that I was having some trouble reading freeway signs from a distance and thought that strange since my eyeglass prescription hadn't changed much in well over 30 years. I was 46 then. I had also noticed that I got ravenously thirsty after going out for Chinese food and simply could not fit enough water in my stomach to quench the thirst.

So one morning in the clinic where I was training it occurred to me that maybe I should check my blood sugar. My paternal grandfather had had diabetes and took insulin injections, and I had been told early in life that I was fairly likely to get this too since it tended to skip generations. I poked my finger nonchalantly that morning, not expecting anything unusual since my lab work in the past was always pretty normal except for high triglyceride levels. I was absolutely shocked to see the number 453 on the glucose meter! I knew it had to be a mistake so I washed my hands and rechecked. There was no mistake: I was now a diabetic! I sat down and started crying, not something I would ordinarily allow myself to do.

In the next five minutes or so I sat alone and imagined having to be admitted to the hospital, starting to take insulin shots multiple times daily along with poking my finger each time the next shot was due, and, worst of all, losing my pilot's license. I had fallen in love with flying while in high school and had immersed myself in this endeavor, attaining commercial pilot and flight instructor certifications by the age of 19. I'd helped pay my way through college working as an instructor and charter pilot. Next to music and photography, flying was my first love and had obviously become much more than just a hobby. Losing this part of my life seemed truly unbearable. Then I remembered that my grandfather had also gone blind and had one of his feet amputated due to his diabetes. At that moment all hope vanished from my mind and I truly wished I were dead!

Just then Dr. Bob Peterson, my preceptor who was training me in his private practice, walked by and saw me sitting there, clearly not in my usual state of mind. He took me into his office and spent the next 20 minutes or so reassuring me that this wasn't the end of the world for me, that most diabetics could control their disease without insulin shots, that losing weight and exercising would help a lot, that there were pills to treat diabetes, and, most importantly, that I shouldn't have to lose any of my aviation privileges. The relief I felt was indescribable! He also pointed out, however, that this was one of the very worst diseases out there unless it was well managed. That the consequences of not keeping it under control included blindness, kidney failure requiring dialysis treatments several times weekly, amputations of the feet or legs and greatly increased likelihood of heart attacks and strokes. This information was not entirely new to me but the review was very sobering.

Prior to this day I really had no interest whatsoever in the disease we call diabetes. I had already worked over twenty years in my original career as a Clinical Laboratory Scientist which involved testing diabetics and culturing the germs responsible for many of their complications. I found the whole subject of diabetes quite boring. And as I was now transitioning into the actual practice of medicine I intended to specialize in some field where I could pretty much ignore this disease and let others deal with it. Now--like it or not--I was an active player and had no choice but to learn much more and get very involved in "diabetes."

I have learned a lot. I have learned that I really am NOT "diabetic." I have learned that the vast majority of diabetics have what is officially called "type 2 diabetes," which is not diabetes at all but a completely different disease. I have learned that almost all the information available to help inaccurately identified diabetics manage their disease is appropriate only for "type 1 diabetics" which are far fewer in number than those of us who have this other disease.

My intent in writing this book is to *finally* provide a source of information *geared specifically* for you and me, along with the millions of others with this disease and the many millions who have it but don't yet know it. This book is designed primarily to provide *clear guidance* for patients. It is intended to be an oversimplification. It is also intended to provide a resource for medical providers who rarely have the time to explain everything here to each new patient they encounter with this disease. Please read on. And feel free to share this information with friends and family who have also been mislabeled diabetic.

Provider "Apologetics"

To my medical provider and nutrition colleagues: I know that some of the concepts and advice written here will seem controversial or downright outrageous to some of you. I assure you that almost none of this information is unique to my philosophy. There are very few original thoughts presented here. Several of the facts presented here are very different from what you and I were taught many years ago. We were simply taught wrong. No one is at fault. Much has been learned since then but not all new information is quickly accepted. Bear with me. Everything here is true and most useful in getting our "sugar-challenged" patients to goal and keeping them there.

1 What the Heck is CARBOSIS?

Since you're reading this book it is likely that you have been diagnosed with diabetes. If your medical provider (doctor, physician assistant, nurse practitioner) hasn't already told you, the official name for your condition is "type 2 diabetes," which, in my opinion and in the opinions of many other medical professionals and scientists, is a really, really poor choice of names.

Centuries ago it was well known that some people produced very sweet-tasting urine. Pretty gross but true! These same people also tended to urinate a lot and tended to be in poor health generally. Some got very skinny and died quickly while others were obese and lived a bit longer. The sweet urine, however, was universally known to be a bad thing. Eventually this condition was given the name "diabetes mellitus" which was derived from Latin and Greek words and simply implied that the patient "pee'd lots of honey." In those days, of course, no one had a clue as to why this happened to some people and not to others. Nor did they know that the sweet urine, caused by **high blood sugar**, could have **vastly different** causes.

Also many years ago it was observed that some people lost weight steadily and then died, but they never had sweet urine. This was simply called "consumption." We now know that this steady weight loss and death can happen because of **vastly different** reasons such as cancer, tuberculosis, thyroid disorders and so forth.

Nowadays we know that "consumption" is simply a clue to some very specific diseases, some of which can be treated successfully and some can't. We know that a severe sore throat shouldn't simply be called "**throatitis**," but is also simply a clue to some very specific diseases such as strep throat, infectious mononucleosis, cold virus, diphtheria and so forth. Some of these are easily treated and some aren't.

Nonetheless, even in modern times, people who tend to have elevated blood sugar, and/or sugar in the urine, are simply called diabetics. OK, they've actually split this into "type 1" and "type 2," but the causes are as **vastly different** as cancer compared to TB, or diphtheria compared to a simple cold. And the treatments are also **vastly different**. Or should be!

The only disease that should be called diabetes mellitus is **true** diabetes (aka type 1 diabetes). You don't have this. We'll get into that in a bit more detail later.

You have **carbosis**. I should say **we** have **carbosis** because I have it too. Haven't ever seen or heard this word before? That's because I just made it up! Others have called our condition "syndrome X," "metabolic syndrome," "diabesity," and probably several other names I haven't heard of. Most medical providers are familiar with these names but almost no patients have ever heard them and certainly none has stuck in the general vocabulary of laymen's medical terms. I picked *carbosis* out of a long list of ideas because it is simple, easy to remember, and it truly conveys the correct meaning of the disease.

I hope the name *carbosis* sticks because it will be immensely helpful for those who have it, both in defining the problem and in making it easy to treat *correctly and effectively*. (If someone else comes up with a better name that sticks I'll be all for it and it certainly won't hurt my feelings!)

Now let's explore why *carbosis* is NOT diabetes and how this increasingly common but unique medical condition can be controlled/treated successfully with minimal impact on us and our families. You may not even need medication. Blood tests should not be needed more than 2-4 times per year, if that. I'll explain why poking your finger at home to test blood sugar is not only worthless in most cases but is often misleading. I'll explain various other medical problems that need to be monitored also. Let's get started.

2 What You Don't Have

What you don't have is diabetes--that is, *true, type 1* diabetes. True diabetes is a very specific medical problem where the body's own immune system, our defense system against infection, goes haywire and starts attacking our own tissues. Diseases such as this one are called *autoimmune* and include other conditions such as thyroid problems, psoriasis, lupus and rheumatoid arthritis. In this case the target tissue is the part of the pancreas that produces insulin, called beta cells. We are born with fully functioning beta cells that produce all the insulin we need for normal functioning. But these cells can be destroyed fairly quickly, leaving a person completely dependent on insulin shots.

Insulin is a special hormone that acts as the gatekeeper to allow glucose, a sugar that is the substance our bodies use mainly for fuel, to enter our cells, especially the muscle cells. Without insulin, the glucose can't get inside the cells that need it for fuel. When this happens, the glucose simply builds up in the blood stream causing higher and higher blood sugar levels while the rest of the body literally starves. There are other hormones produced in the small and large intestines that also play a big part in regulating blood sugar, but insulin is the main player here.

In true diabetics, the pancreas loses the ability to make insulin. Left untreated, these people lose weight rapidly and starve to death. They must take insulin shots multiple times each day in order to stay alive. They also must eat some carbohydrates (starches and sugars). Their blood sugar tends to fluctuate wildly which leads to many related problems. This condition is far less common than carbosis. It tends to start in childhood and is usually treated by endocrinologists, who specialize in endocrine disorders.

Unfortunately most of the literature you'll find about diabetes applies quite well to this **true, type 1** diabetes, but does not help us much in understanding or treating the much more common condition that you and I have, **carbosis**.

3 What You Do Have

What you do have is a very different condition. The vast majority of people with blood sugar problems have **carbosis**. This word simply means "problems with carbohydrates."

The word "carbohydrate" is a chemical term that refers to sugars and starches. Why starch? Because a molecule of starch is simply a long chain, or cluster of chains, of sugar molecules hooked together. Starch is really pure sugar in concentrated form; it just doesn't taste sweet like most sugars do. Our taste buds recognize the *shape* of molecules and don't register a sweet sensation when sugar is encountered in chains or clusters.

See the following illustrations:

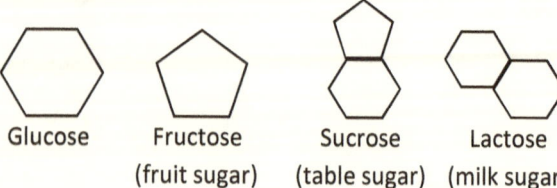

Glucose   Fructose   Sucrose   Lactose
           (fruit sugar) (table sugar) (milk sugar)

Starches

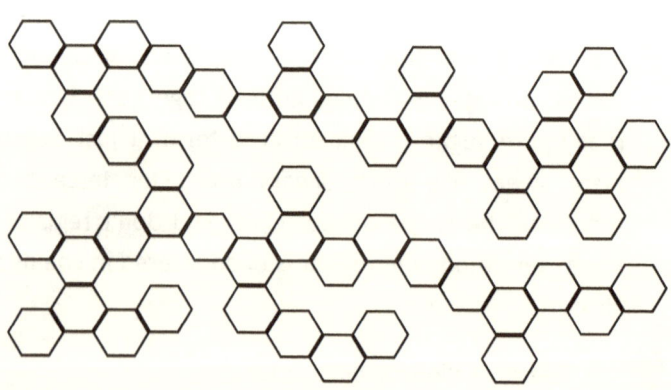

A person with carbosis can be called "carbotic," just like those with diabetes are called diabetic. We carbotics produce plenty of insulin in most cases. In fact, early on we tend to produce too much insulin. The root of our problem is that our cells, primarily the muscle cells, have become resistant to our own insulin. So the pancreas simply makes more and more insulin, trying to keep our blood sugars as normal as possible. This condition takes years to develop and there are no obvious symptoms so most people with carbosis don't even know they have it. Yet.

Simply put, we cannot process carbohydrates correctly, so we eventually develop elevated blood sugar levels, especially after meals. In a nutshell, carbohydrates are *quite toxic* to us whereas they may be less so for normal people. Just as peanuts, shellfish, alcohol and other substances can be quite toxic to some people and less so for others. Remember, *toxic* means **poisonous**!

I want you to stop right here and read the upcoming sentence carefully. You'll see it over and over again because it is the most important part of this manual:

The single most important thing to do to manage carbosis is to avoid eating carbohydrates.

4 Why Carbosis is Such a Bad Thing

The consequences of having abnormally elevated blood sugar long-term are horrible! High blood sugar causes gradual but *irreversible damage* to the *eyes*, the *kidneys*, the *nerves* and the entire *circulatory system* including the *heart*.

Imagine yourself sitting in a wheelchair with dark glasses, a red-and-white cane, stumps where your legs used to be with tubes running your blood through a dialysis machine three times a week for hours just to stay alive. No kidding! There are millions of people who fit that picture exactly. Because they chose to ignore the fact that carbohydrates are poisonous to them! Or, possibly, because no one clearly explained this to them. The majority of people with uncontrolled blood sugar eventually die of heart disease compounded by kidney failure.

Take a good long look at the following illustration. Imagine yourself as this person. Think of your children or grandchildren and of how being in this predicament would affect your interactions with them.

Feel free to make a copy of this illustration and hang it on your refrigerator or bathroom mirror. You can even paste a picture of your own face in the appropriate place for added effect.

Dialysis centers are the fastest growing segment of the medical industry. They are already the single biggest expense to the Medicare Program.

And it is so easy to avoid these problems! Just by making a few simple changes in your diet to keep your blood sugar in control.

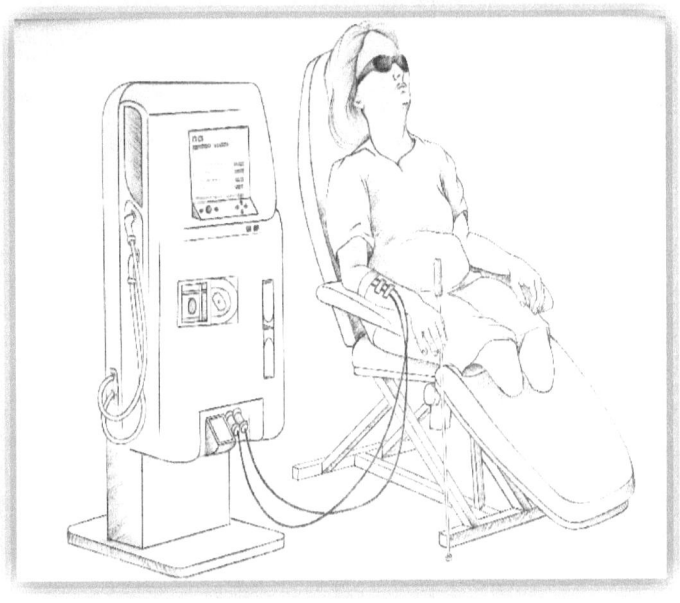

Let's call this person "Blood-sugar Blanche"

B – Blind
L – Legs amputated
A – Atherosclerotic
N – Nerve problems
C – Circulatory problems
H – Heart disease
E – Existing only because of dialysis treatments

Daryl Wein

Notes

5 How to Know If You Have Carbosis

First let's talk about some of the most common clues. Carbosis is highly genetic. If others in your family or of your racial history have blood sugar problems, you are much more likely to have this also.

Carbosis is usually associated with obesity. (Whether the obesity is the cause of carbosis or carbosis is the cause of the obesity is not entirely clear.)

The majority of people with carbosis also have elevated blood pressure. Normal blood pressure while at rest is considered to be 140/90 or lower most of the time.

Another reliable clue is abnormal elevation of triglycerides in the blood, especially if the level of HDL cholesterol (the good cholesterol) is low. In fact, if the amount of triglycerides is more than five times the amount of HDL cholesterol, you most likely already have some resistance to your own insulin, even if your fasting blood sugar appears normal. Blood sugar after meals is often abnormally elevated. This condition can be called *pre-carbosis*.

Two clues to fully-developed carbosis are excessive thirst after eating high-carbohydrate meals and a gradual but steady change in vision. When the blood sugar is high enough (over 300), it actually causes the corneas to swell some and this in turn alters the vision.

There is a brand new test (only three prototype instruments in the country as of this writing) that measures sugar attached to protein in the lens of the eye. This test can be done in less than 3 minutes and is 95% accurate in detecting the presence of abnormally high blood sugar. Ask your local optometrist.

If you have even one of these tell-tale signs, you should ask your medical provider to test your blood. The first test to do, if not already done, is a fasting lipid panel and glucose (nothing but water for at least 12 hours). The lipid panel should include triglycerides, total cholesterol, LDL and HDL cholesterol levels and "non-HDL" cholesterol. The most important finding here is the ratio of triglyceride to HDL cholesterol being more than 5. The non-HDL cholesterol doesn't help with the diagnosis of carbosis but will be very important to know for other reasons. More on this later.

A glucose tolerance test is a procedure where the fasting blood sugar is checked and then an oral dose of glucose is administered, usually in liquid form. The blood sugar is then rechecked periodically. This is a fairly antiquated test but there are a few situations where it can still be used appropriately.

The supreme test of all tests for blood sugar, however, is the hemoglobin A1C, or A1C for short. I don't use this test for general screening but if *any* of the above clues exist it is warranted in my opinion. This test actually shows what a person's blood sugar has averaged, minute by minute, over the last 3-4 months. It accounts for every meal, every snack, every skipped meal and every overindulgence. (And you thought no one was watching!)

The normal range for A1C for most labs is about 4.0 – 5.8. If you're in this range you don't have carbosis. Yet. If you have any of the above clues, check again in a year, sooner if you start getting extra thirsty after meals.

If your A1C is 5.9 – 6.2 you likely have pre-carbosis and should start the maintenance steps outlined later for full-blown carbosis.

If your A1C is over 6.2 you clearly have carbosis but are probably in the early stages. You should immediately start the maintenance steps outlined later.

If your A1C is more than 6.5 don't stop reading until you have at least finished **Chapter 7**!

Daryl Wein

Notes

6 How to Manage Carbosis to Avoid All the Bad Stuff!

The single most important thing to do to manage carbosis is to avoid eating carbohydrates.

I can't emphasize this enough.   Remember, carbohydrates are **_poison_** to those of us with carbosis!

The body does need fuel to operate, and glucose (sugar) is the fuel that's used primarily. But your body can, and will, make all the fuel you need from the protein and fat in your diet. **_There is no need to consume any sugars or starches at all_**.

Once you consume carbohydrate you're stuck with it. Your insulin, if effective, will allow it to move into your muscle cells. You must then move those muscles to use it up or it simply gets sent back to the liver to be converted to fat and stored. Your heart, diaphragm, gut muscles and nervous system will, of course, use some, but the rest just goes into storage. You simply get fatter! People think that insulin *gets rid of high blood sugar*. It doesn't. It just helps move it from place to place. Almost all other non-insulin medications do the same thing.

Keeping the A1C under 6.5 (under 7.0 for those who take insulin shots) is the goal. If you do this you can rest assured that none of the bad stuff previously described is likely to happen to you.

For those with A1C which is elevated *at all*, you should consider this: **Each 1.0 point reduction in your A1C decreases your likelihood of getting *any and all* of the complications described in Chapter 4 by about 40%. Another way to look at this: *each* 1.0 point *increase* almost doubles your likelihood of complications!**

Diet, weight loss and exercise are the big three for managing carbosis. Diet is the most important of these and we'll get into more specifics on this topic in the next chapter.

There are a number of medications available to *help* with blood sugar control but *none that will control this problem by itself*. Most carbotics can control the excess blood sugar 75-100% *just by following a very low-carbohydrate diet*.

See the following example:

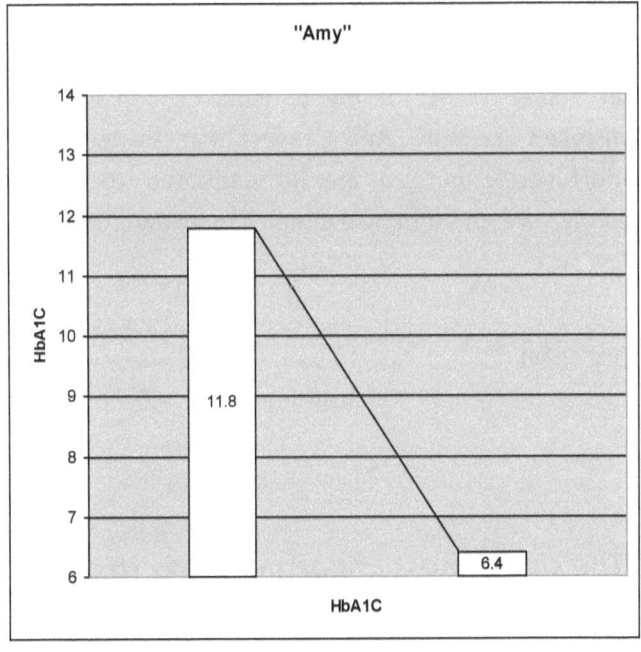

(Examples are all real people; names have been changed for privacy reasons.)

Amy was sent to me from her gynecologic nurse practitioner who discovered high blood sugar from a random fingerstick check. Her NP had her get the A1C checked and it was 11.8. We had a lengthy visit discussing diet through an interpreter and she clearly took my advice to heart. The A1C check 3 months later was 6.4 as you can see. She had also lost 16 pounds just from avoiding the carbohydrates. Remember, this result is from *diet reform alone*!

Amy is the *poster child* patient that I see so often! I wish I could *copy & paste* her story onto every carbotic that I see. Most of my patients do remain well-controlled like this. And I expect that Amy will also. Unfortunately not all are so dedicated to staying healthy. Watch for more examples to follow . . .

Once again . . .

The single most important thing to do to manage carbosis is to avoid eating carbohydrates.

7 Daily Maintenance - The Short Lists

This is where the rubber meets the road so to speak. This chapter deals with the specifics of what to eat and what not to eat in order to keep your blood sugar controlled, which means you can avoid all the bad consequences described earlier. The first Short List includes the most common *high carbohydrate* foods that people eat. The second consists of common foods lowest in carbohydrates.

Remember:

The single most important thing to do to manage carbosis is to avoid eating carbohydrates.

Short List A – The BAD STUFF - DON'T EAT THESE!

Sugary Foods

- All desserts, candies, ice cream, cakes, pies, cookies, sodas - the obvious stuff

- All fruits and fruit juices - some fruits are worse than others, bananas are worst

- Milk & yogurt - these have lactose which is less sweet than other sugars

Starchy Foods

- All breakfast cereals - even oatmeal is mostly starch

- All breads, and everything else made from flour - pasta, noodles, crackers, bagels, pancakes, etc.

- Rice - almost pure starch

- Potatoes - quite high in starch.

- Corn - actually high in both starch and sugar

- Tortillas - both kinds (flour or corn)

- All chips or crackers

Short List B - The IDEAL DIET FOR CARBOSIS

<u>The Foods Lowest in Carbohydrates</u>

- Eggs - fixed any way you like them

- Cheeses of any kind - firmer cheeses are the lowest

- Meats of any kind - the only exception to this is liver

- Fish of any kind, and most shellfish - just not breaded or battered

- Green salads - avoid croutons, use tomatoes in moderation

- Green vegetables, cauliflower, summer squashes (zucchini, yellow crookneck, etc.)

- Nuts and beans - in moderation

- Condiments such as regular mayonnaise, mustard, butter - no carbs in these

- Any sugar-free beverages - water, Crystal Light, tea, diet sodas, etc.

- Pork rinds - this is the ONLY crunchy snack I know of that has no carbs

See Appendix A and Appendix B for much more comprehensive lists of foods and their respective carbohydrate contents.

This data is provided by the U.S. Department of Agriculture (USDA).

Appendix A is sorted by carbohydrate content, highest to lowest.

Appendix B is an alphabetical listing to make it easy for you to look up specific food items.

Once you know how your A1C tests are running it is reasonable to add some of the other lower carb foods to your diet – as long as the A1C continues to remain less than 6.5. If it starts to creap upwards you need to go back to the short list foods only. The other alternative, of course, is to add medication as needed.

8 Medication

If we really *must* add medication(s), we should discuss the various options available. A general rule-of-thumb is that each medication is likely to lower the A1C by about 1.0 point.

The first choice for medications to add is always Metformin (Glucophage, etc.). This is usually well-tolerated but can cause diarrhea or upset stomach. It also interferes with medicine used for general anesthesia so must be stopped prior to surgery.

Why Metformin is always the first choice remains somewhat of a mystery to me. My guess is simply tradition. I have heard that it decreases the likelihood of cancer and heart disease somewhat and may help a little with weight loss.

The next step, if we really *must,* would be to add your medical provider's choice of any one or more of the following drugs (don't even try to pronounce most of these names!):

A TZD (thiazolidinedione) such as **Actos** (pioglitazone) or **Avandia** (rosiglitazone)

A GLP-1 agonist such as **Byetta** (exenatide), **Victoza** (liraglutide) or **Bydureon** (exenatide extended-release), or a DPP-4 inhibitor such as **Januvia** (sitagliptin), **Onglyza** (saxagliptin), **Tradjenta** (linagliptin), **Nesina** (alogliptin).

A SGLT2 inhibitor such as **Invokana** (canagliflozin, the only one of its kind as of this writing)

There are a few other older medications but these are rarely used nowadays.

Medications of last resort

A *nearly last resort* option if all else has failed so far to get the blood sugar under control is a class of old medications called sulfonylureas or SU's (glipizide, glyburide, glymepiride). I thoroughly despise these medications because I'm convinced that they are not nice to the pancreas!

As mentioned earlier, most of us with carbosis are

producing an overabundance of insulin. In other words, the pancreas is already "huffing and puffing," trying to crank out enough insulin to offset the resistance we have developed to our own insulin. Guess what these medications do? They simply *force* the overworked pancreas to crank out *even more* insulin! The mental picture this gives me is of an old work horse faithfully plowing the field while the farmer beats it mercilessly with a whip. How long do you think the pancreas is going to hold up under these conditions?

This type of medication is also famous for making the blood sugar plunge way too low at times (hypoglycemic episodes) which is not only very uncomfortable but dangerous. And what do people do when their blood sugar is too low? They eat or drink sugar! Poison! This makes them feel much better quickly, of course, but the sugar level goes up and down like riding a teeter-totter. I picture this like trying to drive your car with one foot firmly planted on the brake. Something's going to go wrong here!

There is one SU-like medication class, meglitinides, that deserves honorable mention. It includes Starlix (nateglinide) and Prandin (repaglinide). These medications are taken only before meals and gently nudge the pancreas to crank out a little extra insulin, just for this meal. It is sometimes appropriate for patients who are almost under control, but who just need a little extra help. I have two patients on these as of this writing.

The *very last resort*, in my opinion, is insulin shots.

But it is a fact that some carbotics eventually lose the ability to produce enough insulin to manage their carbohydrate intake even if it is minimal. This is usually caused by years of neglect or denial, or long-term use of the sulfonylurea drugs described above.

At this point the carbotic becomes fairly like the true diabetic in that they become dependent on insulin shots for the remainder of their lives. Insulin can be nasty stuff! It is tricky. It is like riding a giant roller coaster. Your blood sugar is either too high or too low much of the time. And insulin can make the blood sugar drop so low, so suddenly, that it can be fatal. It is nearly impossible to keep the blood sugar stable. People are constantly adjusting the amount of insulin they take, and/or the amount of sugar they consume. For this reason an A1C level of 7.0 is considered to be as good as we dare shoot for. Any lower and we know that the sugar level is going too low too often to be safe.

See the following illustrations and examples:

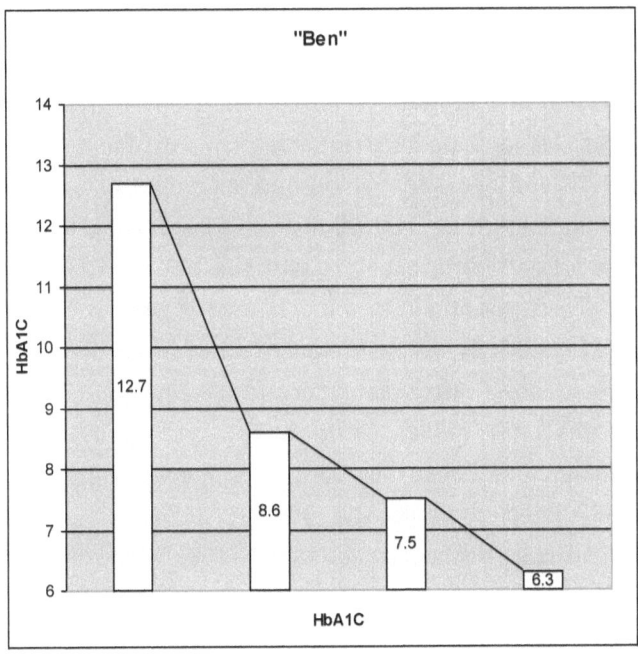

Ben came to see me several years ago as a new patient and hadn't seen a doctor for many years. He did have a family history of "diabetes" and had been steadily gaining weight for a number of years. As is often the case with us men, his wife finally convinced him to get a check-up. He complained that he seemed to get very thirsty after meals, especially after spaghetti and sourdough bread, his favorites (mine too!). He was 43 at the time and about 80 pounds overweight.

His initial screening blood tests were OK except for very high triglycerides over 800 (normal under 150), low HDL cholesterol and fasting glucose of 136 (normal under 100). This is classic for carbosis. My guess is that he had had it for at least a year or two.

After finding that his A1C was 12.7 we had the long talk about diet and what can happen if this isn't controlled and he took it seriously. His dad was on dialysis and had already had one leg amputated so my warnings were already familiar to him. I started him right off on Metformin along with the diet.

Three months later his A1C had improved to 8.6. He insisted that he was following the diet consistently, so we added Actos as a second medication. Three months later it was down to 7.5 and he was still following the diet so we added Byetta, a fairly new non-insulin injected medication. As you can see, we got his A1C to 6.3. His sugar has remained well-controlled so far and he has lost over 40 pounds.

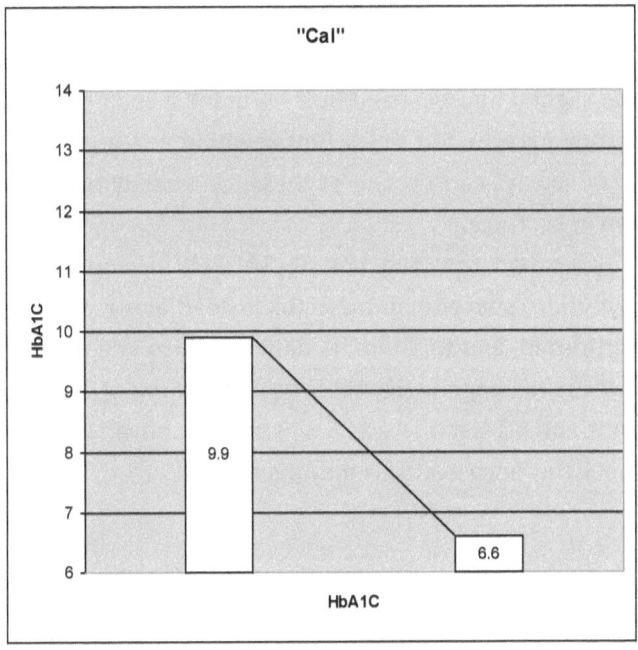

Cal recently had a change in his insurance and transferred to my care as a result since he could no longer go to his long-term regular provider. He had been diagnosed with "diabetes" about five years prior and was already taking Metformin and Glyburide (Ugh!). He hadn't had lab work in well over two years. He was in his mid 50's and quite overweight. His initial A1C at my clinic was 9.9.

He had been told to stop drinking regular sodas and to avoid candy bars, and he usually followed this advice. Otherwise he had been given no other specific dietary advice.

He had noticed that often an hour or two after taking his Glyburide he felt shaky, sweaty, fuzzy-headed and slightly nauseated. But if he drank a soda or some orange juice he felt much better within a few minutes. So he always carried one of these, or a candy bar, with him in his truck.

We had the long talk about diet. I stopped his Glyburide, started him on Actos instead along with the Metformin, and told him he didn't need to keep poking holes in his finger. His A1C's have been under 7.0 ever since and his last one was 6.6 as shown above. We only check this once every six months now.

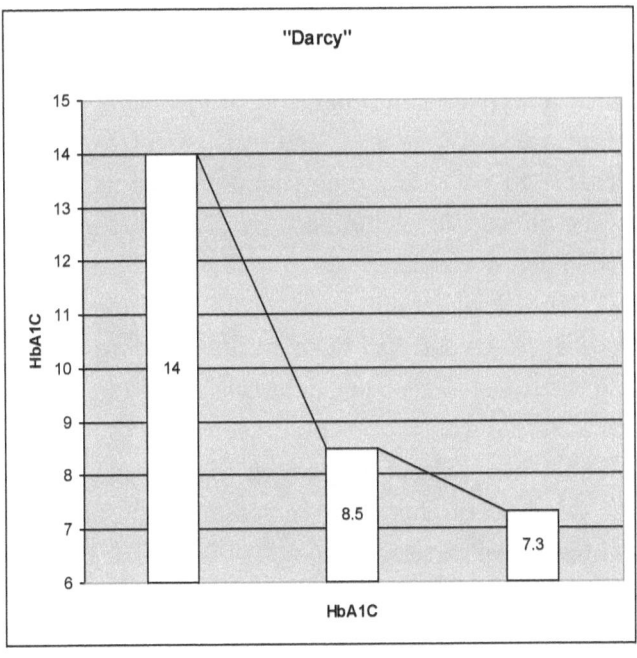

Darcy is another new patient for me, was diagnosed with "diabetes" 10 years ago and recently lost her job. She is now on Medicaid and has had to switch from her private practitioner to the government-funded clinic where I work part of the time. She had been taking Metformin, Actos and Januvia but has been out of these medications for a couple of months. She hasn't had a blood test in over a year. She has never had any dietary advice except for "avoid sweets." Turns out she has quite a sweet tooth and hasn't been heading this advice at all. Her initial A1C here was 14.

We, of course, had a *very* lengthy discussion about diet. She got my hand-written copies of "The Short Lists," and her Metformin and Actos were refilled. These are both generic and are therefore readily available to her. Any other name-brand medications will be difficult to obtain because of her government-funded pharmacy plan.

Her A1C did come down to 8.5 in the next three months. Since she had been so out of control for so long, I suspected that her beta cells were too burned out to respond to further oral medication so I started her on a low dose of long-acting "basal insulin." Her A1C was 7.3 last check, so I increased her insulin dose slightly. If we can keep her A1C about 7.0 she should still avoid the worst of the possible consequences.

The last example is my greatest source of frustration! Meet Evelyn:

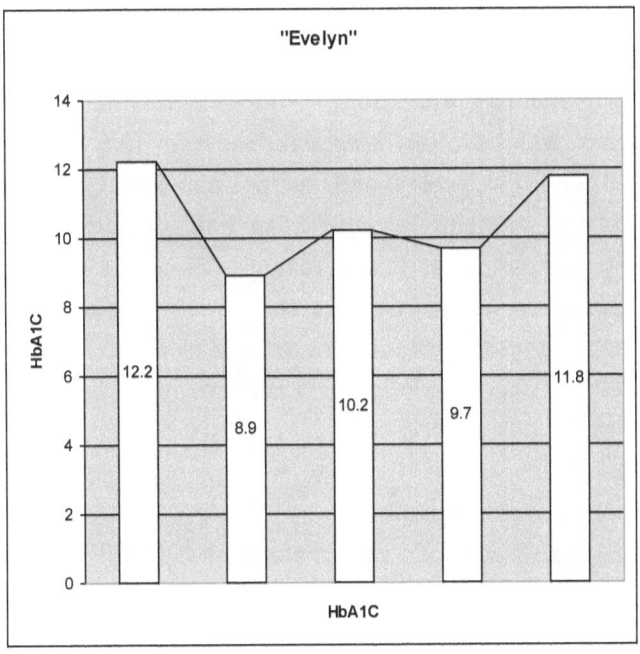

Evelyn has had carbosis for about 10 years. Over and over she's heard the long talk about diet and the consequences of not getting and keeping her blood sugar under control. She has been on and off all the different oral medications out there. If the co-pay is more than $10, she simply stops when the samples run out. She earns too much to qualify for patient assistance programs where medications can be gotten at no cost. She's not willing to try anything that has to be injected, insulin or not.

Honestly I never really know what she's taking, if anything, to help with her carbosis. It is clear that she has made very little effort, if any, to modify her diet to avoid carbohydrates. (Her granddaughter tells me she still likes her ice cream and regular sodas!)

Her husband recently woke her up complaining that she had a very sharp toenail. Turns out she had stepped on a small nail and the point was protruding out the top of her foot between the toes! She has no feeling in her feet. She gets laser treatments on her eyes periodically and can no longer see well enough to pass a driver test. Blood tests show her kidneys are only functioning at 30%.

She is what we call in medicine a "train wreck." She is slowly dying but won't listen. Or doesn't care. She will become exactly like "Blanche" within the next few years. And all she really needed was to change her diet a little in the first place! She could have remained perfectly healthy. Her family will miss her. What a tragedy!

Another reminder is in order here:

The single most important thing to do to manage carbosis is to avoid eating carbohydrates.

9 Preventive Maintenance

Just like your car, you need to have a plan to provide preventive maintenance for your carbotic body.

<u>Blood Sugar</u>

The way we monitor blood sugar best is to have the A1C test done *every 3 months*. If your blood sugar is well controlled and has been consistently well controlled for quite a while, it is completely appropriate to back this off to every 6 months.

In regards to daily fingerstick blood sugar checks, I am convinced, as many others are, that this is usually a waste of time and money for those of us with carbosis. It is only necessary when taking insulin shots. I discourage my carbotic patients from doing this as it is not only unnecessary but often gives them a false sense of security - they see a number that *isn't too bad* and are tempted to eat something they shouldn't. I haven't poked a hole in my finger (intentionally) for over 14 years as of this writing.

Blood Pressure & Kidneys

As mentioned earlier, many people with carbosis also have elevated blood pressure, called hypertension. And also mentioned earlier is the dreaded complication of uncontrolled blood sugar - kidney failure. And, by the way, high blood pressure is the other thing besides blood sugar that leads to kidney failure. Quite conveniently there is a class (two closely related classes really) of blood pressure medications that are also used to help protect the kidneys from the effects of high blood sugar. These are called ACE inhibitors or ACEI's (lisinopril, enalopril, benazepril, anything that ends with "-pril") and Angotensin Receptor Blockers or ARB's (Cozaar, Diovan, Micardis, Avapro, Benicar, Atacand, Teveten; their generic names all end with "-sartan").

I believe that all of us with carbosis can benefit from taking one of these medications for prevention. If you have high blood pressure you will likely need the higher doses and may take these in conjunction with additional blood pressure medications, if needed, to keep hypertension under control.

An *annual urine test* called microalbumin is necessary in all carbotics to monitor for the earliest signs of kidney damage so that, if present, it can be treated aggressively to prevent kidney failure.

Cholesterol & heart disease

As mentioned earlier, nearly all carbotics have abnormal lipids, that is triglycerides, total cholesterol, LDL and HDL cholesterol and Non-HDL cholesterol. This is mainly genetic. The elevated triglycerides will almost always be dramatically improved with the low-carb diet. This will also improve the low HDL cholesterol some. But LDL cholesterol, the bad guy responsible for heart attacks and strokes, is hardly affected at all by diet. More on this in a separate chapter.

I believe that all of us with carbosis will benefit from taking cholesterol-lowering medication regardless of our LDL and Non-HDL cholesterol levels. Certainly if the LDL cholesterol is more than 100 or the Non-HDL cholesterol is more than 120 we would be *foolish* not to take medication.

My favorite cholesterol-lowering medication, especially now that it is generic, is Lipitor (atorvastatin). There are many other options available depending on how bad your lipid situation is. I have been taking two different types of cholesterol-lowering medications for years because my lipids are particularly bad when untreated.

An *annual fasting lipid panel* is a must for those of us with carbosis to monitor and treat lipid problems to prevent heart disease. Remember that most carbotics who are poorly controlled eventually die of heart attack.

Eyes

An *annual dilated eye exam* by an ophthalmologist or retinal specialist is imperative. Eye damage from high blood sugar is most likely to show up within the first five years of having carbosis but in some cases may not develop until later. If necessary, laser treatments of the retina may be used to limit damage. Remember, most carbotics have it for years before being diagnosed.

Feet & Nerves

Many carbotics develop numbness of the toes and feet. This can begin years before they even know they have carbosis. It is, unfortunately, usually irreversible. If severe, it can leave the feet vulnerable to injury without even knowing. In these cases the feet should be checked regularly for sores, cuts, ulcers or other signs of infection including nail fungus which is only a cosmetic problem for those without carbosis. Since the blood circulation is also compromised in people with uncontrolled blood sugar, infections of the feet usually require special effort to eradicate. Don't neglect your feet!

Another nerve problem involving the feet is "peripheral neuralgia," a common problem in carbotics where the feet and lower legs have burning pain in addition to numbness. There are several medications that can help with this condition. Peripheral neuralgia is not limited to carbotics as we see it in other people as well. It is particularly common in people who consume alcohol in excess.

Other nerves can be affected in carbotics including the nerves that control the muscles in the stomach and intestines. Multiple nerve abnormalities should be addressed by a neurologist, a specialist in problems of the nervous system.

10 A Few Tips on Weight Loss and Exercise

I have great news for you! The dietary guide given in Chapter 7 is precisely the most helpful advice you'll need for weight loss also. If you plan to make a concerted effort to lose weight your best bet is to *aim for zero* carbohydrates in your diet. The closer you can get to zero the more weight you will lose. Even the small amount of starch found in a single soda cracker will likely stop weight loss in most overweight people for about 24 hours.

Insulin is fattening. Insulin production from the pancreas is stimulated whenever we consume any digestible carbohydrate. Those of us with carbosis already have high insulin levels, usually. Besides allowing glucose (and potassium) to get into our cells, insulin is also responsible for storing fat in our fat cells. Fat cannot get stored without insulin. *The lower the insulin level the less fat stored.*

Exercise will always help with weight loss, but the most important factor, by far, is the diet. Exercise of any kind will do. There is a common misconception that if you want to lose weight from the abdomen you must exercise the abdominal muscles. From the legs it's the leg muscles. And so forth. This is a myth. Where fat tends to build up is strictly genetic. Any exercise will help equally throughout the body. Low-impact exercise such as power-walking or swimming are great and are much nicer to the joints than running or jogging.

11 Extra Info on Lipids

The word "lipids" refers to fats, cholesterol and triglycerides. Like carbohydrates, fats are long chains of smaller molecules, called fatty acids, hooked together. When we digest fat, the liver converts the fat into triglycerides which are shorter chains of three fatty acids. An excess of triglycerides circulating in the blood is a risk factor for heart problems in addition to the cholesterol we've all heard about.

The most common cause for elevated triglycerides in the blood is insulin resistance, the primary cause of carbosis. Just eliminating carbohydrates from the diet usually has a dramatic effect on lowering triglycerides. Elevated triglycerides can also be caused by alcoholism, pancreatitis and some genetic disorders.

Cholesterol found in the blood is carried around as "lipoprotein" *particles.* These particles are literally microscopic lumps of protein with cholesterol and triglycerides mixed in together. There are several different classes of these particles but we'll only discuss the main two here: LDL and HDL. These particles can be either good or bad for the heart: LDL (low-density lipoprotein) is the worst and is the main cause of coronary artery disease/heart attacks, arteriosclerosis, strokes and PAD (peripheral artery disease).

Interestingly, LDL can be found in different sizes and it is the *small* LDL particles that cause all the problems. Larger LDL particles cannot get into the areas between and behind the cells which line the arteries so they don't cause problems. We've known this for many years but have only recently been able to test the particle sizes routinely.

HDL (high density lipoprotein) is the good stuff that actually collects and removes small LDL particles from the places where they cause problems. HDL particles come in different sizes too but it is the smaller particles that are the most efficient at helping to prevent problems.

The best way to assess these particles is to measure the particle *numbers*. If the *number* of LDL particles is low, this implies that they are either of the larger/healthy variety or there's just not much there. Either is good news. If the number is high you need medication to treat this.

This works for HDL also, just in reverse. If the *number* of HDL particles is high this implies that they are either of the smaller/healthier variety or there is just a lot there, both good news.

12 Extra Info on Sugars and Alternative Fuels

There are a number of different sugars that we encounter in the typical American diet. The two most common are sucrose (table sugar) and high fructose corn syrup (HFCS). These are very similar substances in that they contain about equal amounts of glucose and fructose. Natural sucrose is produced in large amounts in sugar cane and sugar beets. There is enough there to make it profitable to harvest, extract and refine. Sucrose is actually glucose and fructose connected together.

The next most frequent sugars we encounter are fructose and lactose. These are found primarily in fruit and milk, respectively. Lactose is glucose and galactose connected together.

All digestible carbohydrates we consume are quickly broken down primarily into glucose and fructose. Our livers can easily convert proteins into glucose as well. Glucose can also easily be converted into fats.

Glucose in the blood is also what triggers insulin secretion from the pancreas. Remember, we carbotics (most of us) already produce an abundance of insulin. Remember also that insulin is the hormone that causes fat storage in our fat cells. So, the more carbohydrate you consume, the more glucose is produced, the more insulin is secreted and the more fat gets stored! And the fatter we get the more resistant we become to our own insulin! This is a rather nasty vicious cycle.

Fructose is a bit different. The insulin secretion mechanism isn't triggered at all by fructose. But fructose lends itself particularly well to being converted into fat by the liver. And it is also a major player in converting triglycerides into fatty acids to be stored in the fat cells. So fructose is a particularly fattening substance. In fact many scientists are convinced that this is the most fattening substance you can consume! The main sources of fructose are fruit, high-fructose corn syrup and table sugar. And the fruits we have today have been bred for centuries to contain more and more fructose. They are also available in our grocery stores all year long nowadays rather than seasonally.

Just like your car, you must have fuel in order to function, and glucose is the *primary* fuel used to run the body. Also, just like a car, your body can run on alternative fuels. The most common alternative fuel is *ketones* which are produced when we are breaking down fat during weight loss. The brain and nervous system actually works better on ketones than any other fuel but the availability of ketones is usually not sustainable. One exception is found in the traditional Eskimo/Inuit culture where only fat and protein are consumed. These people literally run on ketones along with some glucose that is made by the liver from the fat consumed. They also don't get carbosis. That is unless they start eating carbohydrates!

Another alternative fuel is ethanol which is present in beer, wine, etc. This fuel will *always* interfere with weight loss because, when present, your body will simply stop burning fat and use only the alcohol for fuel until it has been completely used up. So avoid all forms of alcohol when trying to lose weight.

Daryl Wein

Notes

13 Q & A - Questions & Answers

Q: I thought that natural sugar found in fruit was good for you but you are saying it is bad. I don't understand.

A: Sugars and other carbohydrates are fine for thin, non-diabetic, non-carbotic people, and for those who are not trying to lose weight. For the rest of us all carbohydrates are problematic, especially sugars. *Natural* doesn't necessarily mean good! Codeine, morphine and cocaine are natural substances contained in the poppy and coca plants. Natural but deadly.

Q: I have always heard that whole wheat bread is good for you but you have listed bread in the "do not eat" list.

A: 100% whole grain bread is definitely preferable to white bread or cheap "brown bread." But even whole grain bread is mostly starch. It just doesn't digest as quickly because of all the fiber present. If your blood sugars are well-controlled and you are already eating whole grain bread there's no problem. If your A1C is not at goal I'd ditch the breads. Likewise if you are trying to lose weight and having trouble losing I would cut out all breads.

Q: Why can't I simply control my blood sugar with medication? I don't like the idea of having to watch what I eat.

A: You are always in charge of your own body when it comes to deciding whether or not to take medications, follow diets, etc. If you can afford $800+ per month you may actually be able to control your blood sugar with only minimal dietary modification. This means you could be taking up to five different classes of medications, each of which has potential side effects, some of which can be dangerous (think hypoglycemic episodes, kidney or liver problems). Few people I know would opt for this approach.

Q: I thought eggs were high in cholesterol. Don't I have to worry about the high amount of cholesterol in eggs?

A: The cholesterol present in the food we eat has very little to do with the cholesterol found in the blood stream. About 90% of blood cholesterol is actually manufactured by the liver. Eggs are not a problem. Neither are shrimp, beef, etc.

Q: A lot of the foods recommended on the short list are high in fat. Isn't fat bad for you?

A: Not necessarily. The only fats that are known to be harmful are trans-fats which are found in shortening, margarine and any foods containing partially-hydrogenated vegetable oil. We need some fat in the diet to help the liver manufacture a number of important substances including brain and nerve cells as well as the membranes surrounding all the cells in our bodies. Contrary to what most of us have been taught, eating fat does not make you fat. And eating fat has not ever been directly associated with heart disease.

Q: My doctor prescribed a glucose meter and insists that I check my blood sugar every morning. Are you telling me this is not necessary?

A: Yes. That's my opinion. What you and your doctor decide is up to you. Here's the scenario as I see it: You faithfully check and log your sugars every morning before eating, right? Your numbers might run in the 90's or 100's or 120's most of the time. What if you get a 160? Do you do anything different? Of course not (unless you're taking insulin shots). So what have you accomplished by checking? Nothing. There's an unwritten rule in medicine that *you shouldn't order a lab test unless it is likely to cause you to make a change in your treatment of the patient*. The A1C every 3-6 months tells us everything we need to know to treat carbosis. Here's another scenario: You check your morning sugar and find that it is 130. You think "Hey, that's not too bad. In fact, with that number I'm only *barely* diabetic." So you go ahead and eat that apple fritter you've been craving! If you poked your finger 30-60 minutes later you'd be shocked to find it is 400 or so. 'Nuff said.

Q: Would you recommend checking my blood sugar after eating meals instead of first thing in the AM?

A: No. If you eat the *right* stuff your blood sugar will remain pretty constant all the time. If you eat the *wrong* stuff it will go way too high. This is 100 % predictable so why poke a hole in your finger just to confirm what we already know? Checking the A1C every 3 months is as good as it gets for keeping track of your glucose control. Someday we'll all have continuous glucose monitoring and that will be a great thing!

Q: I've seen the term "net carbs" listed on packaged products. What does that mean? Should I pay attention to the total carbs or the net carbs?

A: Great question! The short answer is *only net carbs count*. "Carbohydrate" is a chemical term that refers to the structure and content of a molecule. When we talk about carbohydrates in the diet we're talking about starches and sugars. But there are other carbohydrates that our bodies can't digest. Cellulose is a prime example. Cellulose is the main structural substance in most plants and is technically a carbohydrate. But we lack the enzymes required to break it down into its sugar components. Termites thrive on cellulose. That's why they can consume mostly wood. Cows and other ruminants can also thrive on cellulose because of certain "germs" in their gut that provide the enzymes needed. Another example is the various carbohydrates found in beans. We can only digest about half of these. The other half remain intact until they reach the colon where our friendly bacterial inhabitants are very happy to oblige. They consume these substances with great gusto and cause lots of gas in the process! People with lactose intolerance experience a similar "party" by our friends in the colon.

Q: Some sugar-free foods contain "sugar alcohols." Will these affect my blood sugar or cause me to gain weight?

A: No to both questions. We don't process these substances in a way that will affect blood sugar or cause weight gain or loss. However, some people may experience loose stools when they eat foods containing sugar alcohols. They won't make you drunk either!

Q: I've heard that honey and brown sugar are much better for you because they are more natural and less refined. Is this true?

A: No. Honey is simply sugar with a little water and some flavor variation based on what flowers the bees visited while making the honey. It is still sugar and will cause increased blood sugar and weight gain the same as table sugar. Brown sugar has never been any healthier than white sugar, just less pure. Nowadays brown sugar is made by simply adding a little molasses to white sugar! All bad stuff.

Q: I've seen on TV that oatmeal and other oat cereals are good for you, especially for lowering cholesterol. But the short list says to avoid all breakfast cereals.

A: The short list is correct. Oatmeal and other cereals are fine for thin, non-diabetic, non-carbotic people, and for those who are not trying to lose weight. Otherwise these cereals are just as bad as any other carbohydrates. And oats have never been shown to have any beneficial effect on the heart. Nor any adverse effect. This is just advertising hype.

Q: When I shop for groceries I see low-carb bread, low-carb tortillas, and so forth. Won't these be OK for my blood sugar?

A: The short answer is probably not. It depends. Are you already eating these foods while well controlled (A1C under 6.5)? If so, no problem. If you are having a hard time keeping the A1C where it should be, or if you are trying to lose weight, I wouldn't go there. Remember these are inherently high-carb foods to begin with. Reducing the carbs by even half still leaves them pretty high in carbs.

Q: I've heard that weight loss surgery can actually cure type 2 diabetes. Is this true?

A: So far there is no such thing as a cure for "carbosis." Weight loss will always help. And the Roux-en-Y gastric bypass surgery helps in other ways too. By bypassing the first part of the small intestine there is a powerful effect on gut hormones that can help with blood sugar control immensely, even before the patient has lost any weight. The newer sleeve gastrectomy doesn't have this effect but does have other advantages over Roux-en-Y. The gastric band may help a lot with weight loss (if you don't cheat!) but doesn't have the added advantage of Roux-en-Y.

Q: Friends have told me that brown rice is much better for you than white rice. Do you agree?

A: No. Brown rice still has its original coating of fiber, vitamins and minerals, which are nutritious, but all the starch is still there. White rice is made by polishing this layer away leaving nothing but starch. Some B vitamins are "sprayed" back on to satisfy a government mandate. Brown rice likely digests a bit slower but will eventually yield the same amount of sugar so it is just as harmful to carbotics.

Q: I've heard that you can make imitation mashed potatoes from cauliflower. Have you tried this? Does it taste similar?

A: I've been eating mashed cauliflower for years and it tastes great. The trick is to not add any water. Just add butter and seasoning. Cauliflower has lots of water in it already and can be microwaved just as it is. By the way, you can even make pizza "dough" with cauliflower, cheese and egg that contains almost no carbs. There are many websites with low-carb recipes. Just remember: lower is better. And for weight loss, *aim for zero*.

Q: How about protein shakes or bars? Do you recommend these?

A: Yes. But many have lots of carbohydrate so you have to read all labels carefully. A large department store I know of sells a "weight loss shake" that is loaded with carbs. It will really mess with your blood sugar and will most likely cause weight *gain*. The same store sells a premium protein drink with only two net carbs. This was my lunch every day for nearly three years. Be especially careful with protein bars. Nearly all have carbs. Atkins brand is always reliable but, in my opinion, sometimes a bit pricey.

Q: My mom is always trying to give me sugar-free cookies or sugar-free cakes. Are these safe to eat or will they still affect my blood sugar?

A: "Sugar free" in reference to cookies or cakes is like saying "dehydrated water." There is a relatively small amount of sugar used in most of these recipes but they contain loads of starch which is *pure sugar in concentrated form*. Avoid these!

Q: I always thought milk was good for you because of the calcium. I had no idea it had sugar in it. I really like milk. Are there substitutes without sugar?

A: Milk is a good source of calcium, but cheese is a much better source since almost all of the lactose (milk sugar) is used up in the cheese-making process. Interestingly, with milk, if you remove the fat you end up with an even higher concentration of sugar. Soy and almond milk are both usually much lower in carbohydrates than cow's or goat's milk. But you must always read the labels carefully since manufacturers may add sugar to enhance the taste. Anything to beat the competition!

Q: What's wrong with yogurt? I thought it was good for losing weight.

A: Again, this is advertising hype. You must read labels. Many plain, white, low-fat yogurts still have a lot of sugar. When you add fruit (this isn't fresh fruit either, think fruit jam!) the sugar content goes right up into the small candy bar range.

Q: How about whole wheat pasta? Is this OK for "carbotics?"

A: No. Just like whole wheat bread it is still mostly starch. Read the labels and you'll be amazed at how carbohydrate dense these foods are.

Q: I've read that artificial sweeteners can be just as bad for you as high fructose corn syrup. What is your opinion?

A: I absolutely disagree with this. There is almost no carbohydrate in any of the artificial sweeteners so they can't contribute to elevation of blood sugar or stimulation of insulin secretion.

Q: I see that bananas are described as the worst fruit for carbs. I was told to eat bananas every day for the potassium. Is this wrong?

A: I would have to say yes. Bananas are the "candy bars" of the fruit family! Most people don't need extra potassium unless they take certain medications that deplete potassium (some water pills). If you really do need extra potassium you should be taking pills or liquid potassium. For dietary potassium bananas are actually *way* down the list. Beans and spinach are much better sources of potassium than bananas.

Q: I have read that foods with a low glycemic index are just fine for people with diabetes even though they are high in carbohydrates. Is this true?

A: I would have to disagree with this. The glycemic index for foods gives us an idea of how *quickly* they are likely to cause an increase in blood sugar. The bottom line really is the total carbohydrate content of foods. All digestible carbohydrate will eventually be converted to glucose or fructose.

Q: I have been told that people who go on a low-carbohydrate diet develop ketosis and that this is very dangerous. Do I need to worry about this?

A: No. The condition you're referring to as dangerous is actually *diabetic ketoacidosis*. This is much different from the *ketosis* caused by the low-carb diet. We all have ketosis at various times. Anytime you don't eat for awhile and your body starts burning fat for fuel you will have some ketones in your blood. Ketones are actually a very good fuel for the brain and nervous system. In diabetic ketoacidosis your body is making ketones way too quickly and the buildup becomes toxic. With carbosis this never happens.

Q: I've seen advertisements inviting people to call an 800 number about Actos causing bladder cancer. Hasn't this drug been taken off the market?

A: No, it hasn't, and I hope it never does. Actos does NOT cause bladder cancer. There has been some data that suggests there may be a *miniscule* increase in the number of patients who get bladder cancer who were taking Actos. There is LOTS of evidence that smokers are much more likely to get bladder cancer. Bladder cancer is pretty rare in the first place. If my carbotic patients continue to smoke, and are taking Actos, I simply urge them to quit smoking. I do that anyway. I have taken Actos for years and still do. I prescribe it all the time. These advertisements are placed by the sleaziest of sleazy law firms who file class action lawsuits, then cash in when the drug company offers to settle rather than fight an expensive battle. They get new yachts, new homes, etc., and the people who call their 800 number get pennies at best. You and I get to bear the cost by paying more for medications. These are the Bernie Madoffs of the legal profession!

Q: My family is from Nepal and eating rice is a very important part of our culture. Do I really need to give up rice in my diet?

A: This is a tough one! For people without blood sugar problems rice is just fine. But no matter what your racial history or culture is, if you have carbosis or diabetes, rice is going to cause you lots of problems. Unfortunately many people with cultural diets that are high in carbohydrates are simply given insulin and put on the "roller-coaster." They will all become just like "Blanche" before too long. Many cultures struggle with this issue but I see it as a no-brainer. Don't eat the carbs.

Q: My doctor wants me to start taking insulin shots because my fasting fingerstick blood sugars have jumped up into the 140's. I recently had a cortisone injection in my knee and my orthopedist told me that my sugars would go up. Do I really need to go on insulin?

A: Probably not. I wouldn't. Steroid injections like this only last about three months or so. If, however, you are getting regular epidural steroid shots in your spine and expect to continue this, you probably need to make some sort of change. But simply avoiding the carbohydrates in your diet will probably suffice. Each case is different so do discuss this again with your doctor or other medical practitioner.

Notes

14 Wrap-up

Let's summarize the content of this "Carbosis Owner's Manual & Pocket Guide."

1. Carbosis (aka type 2 diabetes) is very different from true diabetes.

2. The long-term consequences of uncontrolled high blood sugar are *horrible*.

3. All consequences of uncontrolled carbosis are 100% *preventable*.

4. Weight loss and exercise will always *help* to control blood sugar.

5. Medications are often optional but can *help* control blood sugar.

6. And finally, once again:

The single most important thing to do to manage carbosis is to avoid eating carbohydrates.

Or, put more simply: ***Don't eat carbs***!

Notes

Recommendations for Further Reading

There is a wealth of information in print regarding "diabetes" but, as I mentioned in the introduction, nearly all is geared toward true, type 1 diabetes, rather than the carbosis that you and I share. I have read so many books and articles and sat through so many lectures on this subject it makes my head spin, and little applies to carbosis.

In keeping with my intent to provide a manual uniquely brief and concise I will recommend just one author for further reading on this and related subjects. This person is Gary Taubes.

Mr. Taubes, in my opinion, is the greatest investigative science reporter alive today. Through his dogged diligence he has uncovered a treasure trove of previously little-known scientific research on obesity, lipids, heart disease, diabetes, etc. The bulk of this work was done in Europe, especially Germany, prior to WWII. Modern work is finally starting to confirm what was known decades ago but largely ignored.

His two most recent books, "Why We Get Fat and What to Do About It" (2011), and "Good Calories, Bad Calories" (2007) are must reads if you want to learn more on these subjects.

Appendix A

Sorted by Total Carbohydrate

Selected Items From

USDA National Nutrient Database for Standard Reference, Release 25

Content of Selected Foods per Common Measure,
Carbohydrate, by difference (g) sorted by nutrient content

Description	Measure	Carbs (g)
Milk, canned, condensed, sweetened	1 cup	166.46
Pie crust, graham cracker	1 pie shell	155.83
Barley, pearled, raw	1 cup	155.44
Rice, white, long-grain, dry	1 cup	149.65
Tapioca, pearl, dry	1 cup	134.81
Couscous, dry	1 cup	133.95
Dates, deglet noor	1 cup	133.55
Raisins, seedless	1 cup	114.81
Cornmeal, degermed, enriched	1 cup	109.64
Candies, semisweet chocolate	1 cup	107.35
Wheat flour, white, cake, enriched	1 cup	106.90
Bulgur, dry	1 cup	106.22
Candies, white chocolate	1 cup	100.71
Wheat flour, white, bread, enriched	1 cup	99.37
Cornmeal, whole-grain, yellow	1 cup	93.81
Wheat flour, white, all-purpose, self-rising, enriched	1 cup	92.78
Snacks, trail mix, tropical	1 cup	91.84
Wheat flour, whole-grain	1 cup	86.36
Pie crust, standard-type, prepared from recipe, baked	1 pie shell	85.50
Buckwheat flour, whole-groat	1 cup	84.71
Bread crumbs, dry, grated, seasoned	1 cup	82.19
Orange juice, frozen concentrate, unsweetened	6-fl-oz can	81.30
Frybread, made with lard (Navajo)	10-1/2" bread	77.22
Nuts, chestnuts, european, roasted	1 cup	75.73

Description	Measure	Carbs (g)
Rhubarb, frozen, cooked, with sugar	1 cup	74.88
Candies, gumdrops, starch jelly pieces	10 worms	73.19
Grapefruit juice, white, frozen concentrate	6-fl-oz can	71.54
Pie crust, standard-type, frozen, baked	1 pie shell	70.86
Cake, white, with coconut frosting	1 piece	70.78
Fast foods, potato, french fried in vegetable oil	1 large	70.03
Plums, dried (prunes), stewed, no added sugar	1 cup	69.64
Pie, cherry, prepared from recipe	1 piece	69.30
Shake, fast food, chocolate	16 fl oz	68.27
Pie, pecan, commercially prepared	1 piece	67.36
Strawberries, frozen, sweetened, sliced	1 cup	66.10
Snacks, trail mix, regular, with chocolate chips	1 cup	65.55
Raspberries, frozen, red, sweetened	1 cup	65.40
Shake, fast food, vanilla	16 fl oz	65.23
Cookies, graham crackers, plain or honey	1 cup	64.51
Pie, pecan, prepared from recipe	1 piece	63.68
Milk shakes, thick chocolate	10.6 fl oz	63.45
Oat bran, raw	1 cup	62.25
Plums, canned, purple, heavy syrup pack	1 cup	59.96
Peaches, frozen, sliced, sweetened	1 cup	59.95
Fast foods, french toast sticks	5 sticks	58.11
Cake, pineapple upside-down	1 piece	58.08
Pie, apple, prepared from recipe	1 piece	57.51
Plantains, raw	1 medium	57.08

Description	Measure	Carbs (g)
Corn dogs	1 corn dog	55.79
Milk shakes, thick vanilla	11 fl oz	55.56
Beans, white, mature seeds, canned	1 cup	55.54
Apricots, canned, heavy syrup pack, with skin	1 cup	55.39
Submarine sandwich, with tuna salad	6"	55.37
Potatoes, hashed brown, home-prepared	1 cup	54.77
Pie, fried pies, cherry	1 pie	54.53
Sweet potato, canned, vacuum pack	1 cup	53.86
Beans, baked, canned, plain or vegetarian	1 cup	53.70
Beans, baked, canned, with pork and sweet sauce	1 cup	53.36
Pie, lemon meringue, commercially prepared	1 piece	53.34
Peaches, canned, heavy syrup pack	1 cup	52.24
Fast foods, taco with beef, cheese and lettuce	1 large	52.21
Pineapple, canned, heavy syrup pack	1 cup	51.31
Submarine sandwich, with cold cuts	6"	51.05
Pears, canned, heavy syrup pack	1 cup	50.99
Cake, chocolate, without frosting	1 piece	50.73
Blueberries, frozen, sweetened	1 cup	50.49
Pie, lemon meringue, prepared from recipe	1 piece	49.66
Tomato products, canned, paste	1 cup	49.54
Pie, blueberry, prepared from recipe	1 piece	49.25
Bagels, cinnamon-raisin	4" bagel	49.13
Macaroni and cheese, frozen entree	1 package	48.90
Fish sandwich, with tartar sauce and cheese	1 sandwich	48.29
Plantains, cooked	1 cup	47.97

Description	Measure	Carbs (g)
Snacks, pretzels, hard, plain, salted	10 pretzels	47.86
Cheeseburger, double, regular patty and bun	1 sandwich	47.82
Fast foods, sundae, hot fudge	1 sundae	47.67
Beans, navy, mature seeds, cooked, boiled	1 cup	47.41
Beans, baked, with pork and tomato sauce	1 cup	47.29
Bagels, egg	4" bagel	47.17
KELLOGG'S RAISIN BRAN	1 cup	47.15
Fruit cocktail, (peach and pineapple and pear and grape and cherry), canned, heavy syrup	1 cup	46.90
GENERAL MILLS, HONEY NUT CLUSTERS	1 cup	46.86
Pie, cherry, commercially prepared	1 piece	46.57
Corn, sweet, yellow, canned, creamed	1 cup	46.41
KELLOGG'S FROSTED MINI- WHEATS	1 cup	46.39
Shrimp, breaded and fried	6-8 shrimp	45.90
Carbonated beverage, orange	12 fl oz	45.76
Rice, white, long-grain, enriched, cooked	1 cup	45.59
Fast foods, danish pastry, fruit	1 pastry	45.06
Biscuits, plain or buttermilk	4" biscuit	45.05
Chickpeas (garbanzo beans), boiled	1 cup	44.97
Bagels, plain, enriched	4" bagel	44.95
Beans, pinto, mature seeds, cooked, boiled	1 cup	44.84
Rice, brown, long-grain, cooked	1 cup	44.77
Prune juice, canned	1 cup	44.67
Applesauce, canned, sweetened	1 cup	44.60
Coconut, dried (desiccated), sweetened	1 cup	44.33

Description	Measure	Carbs (g)
Barley, pearled, cooked	1 cup	44.31
Submarine sandwich, with roast beef	6"	44.30
GENERAL MILLS, RAISIN NUT BRAN	1 cup	44.28
GENERAL MILLS, BASIC 4	1 cup	43.56
MARS SNACKFOOD US, MILKY WAY Bar	1 bar (2 oz)	43.41
Yogurt, fruit, low fat, per 8 ounce	8-oz	43.24
Macaroni, cooked, enriched	1 cup	43.20
Spaghetti, cooked, enriched	1 cup	43.20
Spaghetti with meat sauce, frozen entree	1 package	43.13
Fast foods, chimichanga, with beef	1 chimi	42.80
Potato, baked, flesh and skin	1 potato	42.72
Cake, white, without frosting	1 piece	42.33
GENERAL MILLS, TOTAL Raisin Bran	1 cup	42.24
Carbonated beverage, grape soda	12 fl oz	41.66
Peas, split, mature seeds, cooked, boiled	1 cup	41.36
Chicken pot pie, frozen entree, prepared	1 small pie	41.21
Pie, pumpkin, prepared from recipe	1 piece	40.92
Pie, blueberry, commercially prepared	1 piece	40.83
Mandarin oranges, canned, light syrup pack	1 cup	40.80
Beans, black, mature seeds, cooked	1 cup	40.78
Candies, marshmallows	1 cup	40.65

Description	Measure	Carbs (g)
Cowpeas (blackeyes), frozen, cooked	1 cup	40.39
Beans, kidney, red, mature seeds, cooked	1 cup	40.36
QUAKER, 100% Natural Granola with Raisins	1/2 cup	40.29
Hamburger; double, large patty; with condiments	1 sandwich	40.27
Noodles, egg, cooked, enriched	1 cup	40.26
Hamburger; single, large patty; with condiments	1 sandwich	40.00
Beans, baked, canned, with franks	1 cup	39.86
Lentils, mature seeds, cooked, boiled	1 cup	39.86
Pie, apple, commercially prepared	1 piece	39.78
Cake, boston cream pie, commercially prepared	1 piece	39.47
Grape drink, canned	8 fl oz	39.38
Lima beans, large, mature seeds, cooked	1 cup	39.25
Carbonated beverage, root beer	12 fl oz	39.22
Grapefruit, sections, canned, light syrup pack	1 cup	39.22
Bagels, cinnamon-raisin	3-1/2" bagel	39.19
Pineapple, canned, juice pack	1 cup	39.09
Clams, breaded and fried	3/4 cup	38.81
Noodles, egg, spinach, cooked, enriched	1 cup	38.80
Chicken fillet sandwich, plain	1 sandwich	38.69
Refried beans, canned, traditional style	1 cup	38.46
Carbonated beverage, pepper-type	12 fl oz	38.27

Description	Measure	Carbs (g)
Plums, canned, purple, juice pack	1 cup	38.18
QUAKER, QUAKER 100% Natural Granola with Oats, Wheat, Honey, and Raisins	1/2 cup	38.08
Pie, chocolate creme, commercially prepared	1 piece	37.97
Beans, kidney, red, canned, solids and liquids	1 cup	37.96
Pie, pumpkin, commercially prepared	1 piece	37.96
Fast Foods, biscuit, with egg and sausage	1 biscuit	37.89
Cake, yellow, with vanilla frosting	1 piece	37.63
Bagels, egg	3-1/2" bagel	37.63
Grape juice, canned or bottled, unsweetened	1 cup	37.37
Beans, great northern, mature seeds, cooked	1 cup	37.33
Carbonated beverage, SPRITE, lemon-lime	12 fl oz	37.32
Spaghetti, whole-wheat, cooked	1 cup	37.16
Potatoes, mashed, whole milk added	1 cup	36.90
Cheeseburger; single, large patty; with condiments and bacon	1 sandwich	36.84
KELLOGG'S POP TARTS, Frosted chocolate fudge	1 pastry	36.61
Couscous, cooked	1 cup	36.46
Cake, gingerbread, prepared from recipe	1 piece	36.41
Cake, sponge, prepared from recipe	1 piece	36.35
Fast foods, nachos, with cheese	6-8 nachos	36.33
Cereals ready-to-eat, wheat, shredded, Plain, sugar and salt free	2 biscuits	36.23
Onion rings, breaded and fried	8-9 rings	36.17

Description	Measure	Carbs (g)
Apricot nectar, canned	1 cup	36.12
French toast with butter	2 slices	36.05
Toaster pastries, fruit (includes apple, blueberry, cherry, strawberry)	1 pastry	36.00
Lima beans, large, canned	1 cup	35.93
Cookies, brownies, commercially prepared	1 brownie	35.78
Cereals, corn grits, white, regular and quick, enriched, cooked with water	1 cup	35.72
Cake, yellow, with chocolate frosting	1 piece	35.43
Carbonated beverage, cola	12 fl oz	35.37
Fast foods, potato, french fried in vegetable oil	1 small	35.22
MARS SNACKFOOD US, SNICKERS Bar	1 bar (2 oz)	35.06
Lima beans, frozen, baby, cooked	1 cup	35.01
Wild rice, cooked	1 cup	35.00
Bananas, raw	1 cup	34.26
Cranberry juice cocktail, bottled	8 fl oz	34.21
Toaster pastries, brown-sugar-cinnamon	1 pastry	34.05
Fast foods, taco with beef, cheese and lettuce	1 small	33.94
Danish pastry, fruit	1 danish	33.94
Pizza, 14" pizza, pepperoni, regular crust	1 slice	33.90
Popcorn, caramel-coated, with peanuts	1 cup	33.89
Cake, chocolate, with chocolate frosting	1 piece	33.82
Bulgur, cooked	1 cup	33.82

Description	Measure	Carbs (g)
Sweet potato, cooked, candied, home-prepared	1 piece	33.73
Buckwheat groats, roasted, cooked	1 cup	33.50
Fast foods, roast beef sandwich, plain	1 sandwich	33.44
Bread, pita, white, enriched	6-1/2" pita	33.42
Papayas, raw	1 papaya	32.89
Lima beans, frozen, fordhook, cooked	1 cup	32.84
Bread, banana, made with margarine	1 slice	32.76
Bread, cornbread, dry mix, prepared	1 piece	32.67
Chickpeas (garbanzo beans)	1 cup	32.38
Pineapple juice, canned, unsweetened	1 cup	32.18
Carbonated beverage, ginger ale	12 fl oz	32.10
Pears, canned, juice pack, solids and liquids	1 cup	32.09
Alcoholic beverage, pina colada	4.5 fl oz	31.95
Grape juice cocktail, frozen concentrate, diluted with 3 volume water	1 cup	31.88
Chocolate-flavor beverage mix, powder, prepared with whole milk	1 cup	31.68
Corn, sweet, yellow, frozen, kernels cut off cob	1 cup	31.65
Cake, shortcake, biscuit-type	1 shortcake	31.53
Milk, chocolate, fluid, lowfat, with added vitamin A and vitamin D	1 cup	31.50
Potatoes, au gratin, dry mix, prepared with water, whole milk and butter	1 cup	31.46
Pie, coconut custard, commercially prepared	1 piece	31.41
Fast foods, hush puppies	5 pieces	31.36

Description	Measure	Carbs (g)
Fast foods, hotdog, with chili	1 sandwich	31.29
Potatoes, scalloped, dry mix, prepared with water, whole milk and butter	1 cup	31.29
Dates, deglet noor	5 dates	31.14
Mangos, raw	1 mango	31.01
Muffins, blueberry (Includes mini- muffins)	1 muffin	30.77
Sweet rolls, cinnamon, with raisins	1 roll	30.54
Milk, chocolate, reduced fat, with added vitamin A and vitamin D	1 cup	30.33
Noodles, chinese, chow mein	1 cup	30.16
Cake, creme-filled, chocolate with frosting	1 cupcake	30.16
Apricots, canned, juice pack, with skin	1 cup	30.11
Rolls, hard (includes kaiser)	1 roll	30.04
Tangerine juice, canned, sweetened	1 cup	29.88
Fast foods, english muffin, with egg, cheese, and canadian bacon	1 muffin	29.69
Fruit punch drink, with added nutrients, canned	8 fl oz	29.69
Tostada, with beans, beef, and cheese	1 tostada	29.66
Malted drink mix, chocolate, powder, prepared	1 cup	29.65
Pineapple and orange juice drink, canned	8 fl oz	29.50
NESTLE, CRUNCH Bar and Dessert Topping	1 bar (1.5 oz)	29.48
Coffeecake, cinnamon with crumb topping	1 piece	29.42
Cake, angelfood, dry mix, prepared	1 piece	29.35
Pears, asian, raw	1 pear	29.29

Description	Measure	Carbs (g)
Chili con carne with beans, canned entree	1 cup	29.08
Milk, canned, evaporated, nonfat, with vitamin A and vitamin D	1 cup	29.06
Burrito, with beans and cheese	1 burrito	29.04
Macaroni and Cheese, canned entree	1 cup	29.03
Muffins, corn, commercially prepared	1 muffin	29.01
Pineapple and grapefruit juice drink, canned	8 fl oz	29.00
Grapes, red or green (Thompson seedless)	1 cup	28.96
Cupcakes, chocolate, with frosting, low-fat	1 cupcake	28.90
Doughnuts, yeast-leavened, glazed, enriched	1 medium	28.76
Orange juice, includes from concentrate	1 cup	28.73
Fast foods, frijoles with cheese	1 cup	28.71
Peaches, canned, juice pack	1 cup	28.69
Danish pastry, cheese	1 pastry	28.69
WHEATENA, cooked with water	1 cup	28.67
Enchilada, with cheese	1 enchilada	28.54
Malted drink mix, prepared with whole milk	1 cup	28.28
Cornbread, made with low fat (2%) milk	1 piece	28.28
Fruit cocktail, (peach and pineapple and pear and grape and cherry)	1 cup	28.11
Oats, regular and quick, cooked with water	1 cup	28.08
KELLOGG'S RICE KRISPIES	1-1/4 cup	28.07
Puddings, chocolate, dry mix, prepared with 2% milk	1/2 cup	28.06

Description	Measure	Carbs (g)
KELLOGG'S CORN POPS	1 cup	28.02
Apple juice, unsweetened	1 cup	28.02
Pasta with meatballs in tomato sauce, canned	1 cup	28.00
Potato salad, home-prepared	1 cup	27.93
Popcorn, caramel-coated, withoutpeanuts	1 cup	27.84
Grapefruit juice, white, canned, sweetened	1 cup	27.83
Puddings, chocolate, dry mix, instant, prepared with 2% milk	1/2 cup	27.77
KELLOGG'S FROSTED FLAKES	3/4 cup	27.65
Potatoes, au gratin, from recipe using butter	1 cup	27.61
Muffins, oat bran	1 muffin	27.53
Applesauce, canned, unsweetened	1 cup	27.50
Orange juice, canned, unsweetened	1 cup	27.41
English muffins, plain, toasted, enriched	1 muffin	27.38
Cake, snack cakes, creme-filled, sponge	1 cake	27.21
Soft-serve ice cream, vanilla, with cone	1 cone	27.15
KIT KAT Wafer Bar	1 bar (1.5 oz)	27.13
Soup, bean with ham, canned, chunky	1 cup	27.12
Bananas, raw	1 banana	26.95
Orange juice, frozen concentrate, unsweetened	1 cup	26.84
Plums, dried (prunes), uncooked	5 prunes	26.83
Biscuits, plain or buttermilk, from recipe	2-1/2" biscuit	26.76

Description	Measure	Carbs (g)
KELLOGG'S COCOA KRISPIES	3/4 cup	26.68
MR. GOODBAR Chocolate Bar	1 bar (1.75 oz)	26.63
Parsnips, cooked	1 cup	26.54
Candies, jellybeans	10 large	26.52
Cake, fruitcake, commercially prepared	1 piece	26.49
KELLOGG'S APPLE JACKS	1 cup	26.46
Danish pastry, cheese	1 danish	26.41
Potatoes, scalloped, home-prepared with butter	1 cup	26.41
CREAM OF WHEAT	1 cup	26.41
GENERAL MILLS, Honey Nut CHEX	3/4 cup	26.25
GENERAL MILLS, Rice CHEX	1-1/4 cup	26.20
Jerusalem-artichokes, raw	1 cup	26.16
Candies, milk chocolate	1 bar (1.5 oz)	26.14
Croissants, butter	1 croissant	26.11
Farina, assorted brands including CREAM OF WHEAT, quick (1-3 minutes)	1 cup	26.10
KELLOGG'S FROOT LOOPS	1 cup	26.01
Puddings, chocolate, ready-to-eat	4 oz	26.00
Puddings, vanilla, prepared with 2% milk	1/2 cup	25.94
Milk, chocolate, whole, with added vitamin A and vitamin D	1 cup	25.85
Lemonade, frozen concentrate, prepared with water	8 fl oz	25.84
Frostings, vanilla, creamy, ready-to-eat	1/12 package	25.80

Description	Measure	Carbs (g)
Orange juice, raw	1 cup	25.79
KELLOGG'S NUTRI-GRAIN Cereal Bars, fruit	1 bar	25.73
GENERAL MILLS, TRIX	1 cup	25.68
Puddings, vanilla, ready-to-eat	4 oz	25.54
GENERAL MILLS, GOLDEN GRAHAMS	3/4 cup	25.53
GENERAL MILLS Corn CHEX	1 cup	25.47
KELLOGG'S RICE KRISPIES TREATS Cereal	3/4 cup	25.41
Croutons, seasoned	1 cup	25.40
Soup, onion, dry, mix	1 packet	25.38
QUAKER OAT CINNAMON LIFE	3/4 cup	25.33
Milk, canned, evaporated, with added vitamin D	1 cup	25.30
Pears, raw	1 pear	25.28
English muffins, plain, (includes sourdough)	1 muffin	25.18
GENERAL MILLS, BERRY BERRY KIX	3/4 cup	25.14
GENERAL MILLS, COCOA PUFFS	1 cup	25.11
Oat bran, cooked	1 cup	25.05
GENERAL MILLS, WHEATIES	1 cup	24.99
REESE'S Peanut Butter Cups	1 package	24.91
KELLOGG'S PRODUCT 19	1 cup	24.90
QUAKER OAT LIFE, plain	3/4 cup	24.88
KELLOGG'S CRISPIX	1 cup	24.85

Description	Measure	Carbs (g)
GENERAL MILLS, KIX	1-1/3 cup	24.85
Mangos, raw	1 cup	24.72
Soup, pea, green, canned, prepared with equal volume water	1 cup	24.70
Waffles, plain, prepared from recipe	1 waffle	24.68
GENERAL MILLS, Wheat CHEX	1 cup	24.66
Muffins, corn, dry mix, prepared	1 muffin	24.55
Puddings, tapioca, ready-to-eat	4 oz	24.51
APPLE CINNAMON CHEERIOS	3/4 cup	24.39
Alcoholic beverage, liqueur, coffee	1.5 fl oz	24.34
Figs, dried, uncooked	2 figs	24.27
GENERAL MILLS, LUCKY CHARMS	1 cup	24.27
Eclairs, custard-filled with chocolate glaze	1 eclair	24.20
Squash, winter, butternut, frozen, cooked	1 cup	24.12
Grapefruit juice , frozen concentrate, unsweetened, diluted with 3 volume water	1 cup	24.03
Frostings, chocolate, creamy, ready-to-eat	1/12 package	24.02
HONEY NUT CHEERIOS	1 cup	23.97
CINNAMON TOAST CRUNCH cereal	3/4 cup	23.92
Peaches, dried, sulfured, uncooked	3 halves	23.92
KELLOGG'S HONEY SMACKS	3/4 cup	23.90
Vegetables, mixed, frozen, cooked	1 cup	23.82
Cocoa mix, powder	3 tsp	23.74

Description	Measure	Carbs (g)
Crackers, matzo, plain	1 matzo	23.73
Fast foods, croissant, with egg, cheese, and bacon	1 croissant	23.65
Cookies, molasses	1 cookie	23.62
Fast foods, taco salad	1-1/2 cups	23.58
KELLOGG, KELLOGG'S Corn Flakes	1 cup	23.55
Snacks, fruit leather, pieces	1 oz	23.48
Malt-o-Meal, plain, prepared with water	1 serving	23.37
Muffins, blueberry, made with low fat (2%) milk	1 muffin	23.20
Fast foods, potatoes, hashed brown	1/2 cup	23.18
QUAKER, CAP'N CRUNCH	3/4 cup	23.09
Sauce, homemade, white, medium	1 cup	22.93
KELLOGG'S ALL-BRAN COMPLETE	3/4 cup	22.91
Potatoes, mashed, dehydrated, prepared from flakes whole milk and butter added	1 cup	22.83
Peas, green, frozen, cooked	1 cup	22.82
Grapefruit juice	1 cup	22.72
GENERAL MILLS, REESE'S PUFFS	3/4 cup	22.68
KELLOGG'S SPECIAL K	1 cup	22.63
Burrito, with beans and beef	1 burrito	22.55
Sherbet, orange	1/2 cup	22.50
Tomato products, canned, puree	1 cup	22.45
GENERAL MILLS, Whole Grain TOTAL	3/4 cup	22.41

Description	Measure	Carbs (g)
CAP'N CRUNCH with CRUNCHBERRIES	3/4 cup	22.33
Tea, instant, sweetened with sugar, lemon-flavored	8 fl oz	22.30
KELLOGG'S ALL-BRAN Original	1/2 cup	22.27
Soup, tomato, canned, prepared with equal volume low fat (2%) milk	1 cup	22.20
Cranberry sauce, canned, sweetened	1 slice	22.17
Bread, white (includes soft bread crumbs)	1 cup	22.08
Rice drink, unsweetened, with added calcium, vitamins A and D	8 fl oz	22.01
Puddings, rice, ready-to-eat	4 oz	22.00
GENERAL MILLS, CHEERIOS	1 cup	21.97
Chili con carne	1 cup	21.94
Apricots, dried, sulfured, uncooked	10 halves	21.92
Potato puffs, frozen, oven-heated	10 puffs	21.92
Carrot juice, canned	1 cup	21.90
Candies, milk chocolate, with almonds	1 bar (1.45 oz)	21.89
Cherries, sour, red, canned, water pack	1 cup	21.81
Candies, gumdrops, starch jelly pieces	10 bears	21.76
Bread stuffing, bread, dry mix, prepared	1/2 cup	21.70
Soup, minestrone, canned, reduced sodium	1 cup	21.69
Watermelon, raw	1 wedge	21.59
Rolls, hamburger or hotdog, plain	1 roll	21.56
Doughnuts, cake-type, plain (includes unsugared, old-fashioned)	1 medium	21.45

Description	Measure	Carbs (g)
CREAM OF WHEAT, plain, prepared with water	1 packet	21.44
Onions, cooked, boiled, drained, without salt	1 cup	21.32
CAP'N CRUNCH'S PEANUT BUTTER CRUNCH	3/4 cup	21.24
GENERAL MILLS, CHEX MIX, traditional flavor	2/3 cup	21.20
Oranges, raw, all commercial varieties	1 cup	21.15
Potato pancakes	1 pancake	21.14
Apples, dried, sulfured, uncooked	5 rings	21.08
Soup, clam chowder, new england	1 cup	21.03
Soup, bean with pork, canned, prepared with equal volume water	1 cup	21.02
Blueberries, raw	1 cup	21.01
Mushrooms, shiitake, cooked	1 cup	20.87
Pie fillings, canned, cherry	1/8 of 21-oz	20.72
Oats, instant, fortified, plain, prepared (boiling water added or microwaved)	1 packet	20.66
Eggnog	1 cup	20.45
Bread crumbs, dry, grated, plain	1 oz	20.41
Cheesecake commercially prepared	1 piece	20.40
Pineapple, raw, all varieties	1 cup	20.34
Tortilla chips, nacho-flavor, reduced fat	1 oz	20.30
Artichokes, (globe or french), cooked	1 cup	20.08
Granola bars, soft, uncoated, chocolate chip	1 bar	19.90
Soybeans, green, cooked	1 cup	19.89

Description	Measure	Carbs (g)
Candies, milk chocolate coated peanuts	10 pieces	19.88
Pizza, meat and vegetable topping, regular crust	1 serving	19.86
Pumpkin, canned, without salt	1 cup	19.82
Chocolate-flavor beverage mix for milk	2-3 tsp	19.63
Peaches, canned, heavy syrup pack	1 half	19.54
Ice creams, vanilla, light	1/2 cup	19.44
Pie fillings, apple, canned	1/8 of 21-oz	19.31
Peas, green (includes baby types), canned	1 cup	19.31
Gelatin desserts, dry mix, prepared with water	1/2 cup	19.16
Bread, egg	1/2" slice	19.12
Ice creams, french vanilla, soft-serve	1/2 cup	19.09
Apples, raw, with skin	1 apple	19.06
Soup, chunky vegetable, canned	1 cup	19.01
Potato chips, reduced fat	1 oz	18.97
French toast, frozen, ready-to-heat	1 slice	18.94
Soup, chicken vegetable, chunky, canned	1 cup	18.89
Muffins, wheat bran, toaster-type with raisins	1 muffin	18.87
Sauce, pasta, spaghetti/marinara	1 cup	18.83
Snacks, granola bars, soft, uncoated, raisin	1 bar	18.82
Ice creams, chocolate	1/2 cup	18.61
Tortilla chips, plain, white corn	1 oz	18.59

Description	Measure	Carbs (g)
Clam chowder, new england, canned, prepared	1 cup	18.50
Lemonade-flavor drink, prepared with water	8 fl oz	18.35
Cake, sponge, commercially prepared	1 shortcake	18.33
Pizza, cheese topping, regular crust	1 serving	18.28
Snacks, granola bars, hard, plain	1 bar	18.26
Beef stew, canned entree	1 cup	18.21
Miso	1 cup	18.20
Squash, winter, all varieties, cooked, baked	1 cup	18.14
Fast foods, hotdog, plain	1 sandwich	18.03
Snacks, fruit leather, rolls	1 large	18.02
Frozen yogurts, chocolate, soft-serve	1/2 cup	17.93
Snacks, corn-based, extruded, chips, plain	1 oz	17.86
Malted drink mix, chocolate	3 tsp	17.77
Cookies, chocolate chip, baked	1 cookie	17.73
KELLOGG'S RICE KRISPIES TREATS	1 bar	17.71
Malted drink mix, natural	4-5 tsp	17.55
Tortilla chips, nacho cheese	1 oz	17.50
Yogurt, plain, skim milk	8-oz	17.43
Frozen yogurts, vanilla, soft-serve	1/2 cup	17.42
Honey	1 tbsp	17.30
Waterchestnuts, chinese, canned	1 cup	17.22

Description	Measure	Carbs (g)
Cookies, oatmeal, regular	1 cookie	17.18
Cake, pound, commercially prepared	1 slice	17.08
Soybeans, mature cooked, boiled, without salt	1 cup	17.08
Beets, cooked, boiled, drained	1 cup	16.93
Sweet rolls, cinnamon, refrigerated dough with frosting, baked	1 roll	16.83
Corn, sweet, white, cooked	1 ear	16.72
Ice creams, vanilla, rich	1/2 cup	16.49
Lime juice, canned or bottled, unsweetened	1 cup	16.46
Tortillas, ready-to-bake or -fry, flour	1 tortilla	16.39
Waffles, plain, frozen, ready -to-heat, toasted	1 waffle	16.27
French toast, made with low fat (2%) milk	1 slice	16.25
Peaches, raw	1 cup	16.22
Cake, angelfood, commercially prepared	1 piece	16.18
Corn, sweet, yellow, cooked	1 ear	16.15
Soup, tomato, canned, prepared with equal volume water	1 cup	16.03
Tostada with guacamole	1 tostada	16.01
Lettuce, iceberg (includes crisphead types)	1 head	16.01
Yogurt, plain, low fat	8-oz	15.98
Candies, carob, unsweetened	1 oz	15.96
Snacks, corn-based, extruded, chips, barbecue-flavor	1 oz	15.93
Chicken, breaded and fried, boneless pieces	6 pieces	15.83

Description	Measure	Carbs (g)
Lemon juice, canned or bottled	1 cup	15.81
Tomatoes, red, ripe, canned, stewed	1 cup	15.78
KELLOGG'S, EGGO, Waffles, Homestyle	1 waffle	15.72
Cookies, brownies, dry mix, special dietary	1 brownie	15.69
Frozen novelties, ice type, italian	1/2 cup	15.66
Bread, pita, white, enriched	4" pita	15.60
Ice creams, vanilla	1/2 cup	15.58
Frozen novelties, fruit and juice bars	1 bar	15.55
Bread, rye	1 slice	15.46
Melons, honeydew, raw	1 cup	15.45
Fish fillet, battered or breaded, and fried	1 fillet	15.44
Oranges, raw, all commercial varieties	1 orange	15.39
Soymilk, original and vanilla, unfortified	1 cup	15.39
Syrups, corn, light	1 tbsp	15.36
Crackers, melba toast, plain	4 pieces	15.32
Bread, pumpernickel	1 slice	15.20
Papayas, raw	1 cup	15.15
Granola bars, soft, milk chocolate coating, peanut butter	1 bar	15.14
Bread, pumpernickel, toasted	1 slice	15.14
Vegetables, mixed, canned	1 cup	15.09
Snacks, corn-based, puffs or twists, cheese-flavor	1 oz	15.03

Description	Measure	Carbs (g)
Soup, chicken vegetable, chunky, reduced fat	1 serving	14.99
Soup, cream of chicken, canned, prepared with equal volume milk	1 cup	14.98
Snacks, potato chips, barbecue-flavor	1 oz	14.97
Onions, raw	1 cup	14.94
Coleslaw, home-prepared	1 cup	14.89
Fast foods, coleslaw	3/4 cup	14.74
Raspberries, raw	1 cup	14.69
Snacks, oriental mix, rice-based	1/4 cup	14.63
Potato chips, sour-cream-and-onion-flavor	1 oz	14.60
Rolls, dinner, plain	1 roll	14.57
Pears, canned, heavy syrup pack	1 half	14.57
Melons, honeydew, raw	1/8 melon	14.54
Peas, edible-podded, frozen	1 cup	14.43
Nectarines, raw	1 nectarine	14.35
Artichokes, (globe or french), cooked	1 medium	14.34
Soup, cream of mushroom, canned, prepared with equal volume low fat (2%) milk	1 cup	14.28
Bread, french or vienna (includes sourdough)	1/2" slice	14.11
Alcoholic beverage, wine, dessert, sweet	3.5 fl oz	14.10
Apples, raw, without skin	1 cup	14.04
Pancakes, plain, dry mix, complete	1 pancake	13.95
Potatoes, french fried, all types	10 strips	13.87

Description	Measure	Carbs (g)
Blackberries, raw	1 cup	13.84
Jams and preserves	1 tbsp	13.77
Cake, pound, commercially prepared	1 piece	13.66
Bread, raisin, toasted, enriched	1 slice	13.66
Pancakes plain, frozen, (includes buttermilk)	1 pancake	13.59
Syrups, maple	1 tbsp	13.41
Cheese sauce, prepared from recipe	1 cup	13.32
Jellies	1 tbsp	13.29
Tomato products, canned, sauce	1 cup	13.18
Fudge, vanilla, prepared-from-recipe	1 piece	13.14
Grapefruit, raw, pink and red, all areas	1/2 grapefruit	13.11
Bread, oatmeal	1 slice	13.10
Melons, cantaloupe, raw	1 cup	13.06
Fudge, chocolate, prepared-from-recipe	1 piece	12.99
Pears, asian, raw	1 pear	12.99
Fudge, chocolate, with nuts	1 piece	12.91
Brussels sprouts, frozen, cooked	1 cup	12.90
Carrots, cooked	1 cup	12.82
MARS SNACKFOOD US, MILKY WAY Bar	1 fun size bar	12.81
Crab, imitation, made from surimi	3 oz	12.75
Strawberries, raw	1 cup	12.75

Description	Measure	Carbs (g)
Bread, rye, toasted	1 slice	12.74
Cheese, ricotta, part skim milk	1 cup	12.64
Alcoholic beverage, beer, regular, all	12 fl oz	12.60
Biscuits, plain or buttermilk, refrigerated dough	2-1/2" biscuit	12.59
Chicken, breast, fried, batter	1/2 breast	12.59
Cereals ready-to-eat, rice, puffed	1 cup	12.57
Bread, cracked-wheat	1 slice	12.38
Bread, whole wheat	1 slice	12.37
Syrups, table blends, pancake	1 tbsp	12.29
Beets, canned, drained solids	1 cup	12.26
Chocolate syrup	1 tbsp	12.21
Milk, lowfat, fluid, 1% milkfat, with added vitamin A and vitamin D	1 cup	12.18
Milk, nonfat, fluid, with added vitamin A and vitamin D (fat free or skim)	1 cup	12.15
M&M's Peanut Chocolate Candies	10 pieces	12.10
Collards, frozen, chopped, cooked	1 cup	12.07
Pumpkin, cooked	1 cup	12.01
Milk, dry, nonfat, instant, with added vitamin A and vitamin D	1/3 cup	12.00
Syrups, chocolate, fudge-type	1 tbsp	11.95
NABISCO SNACKWELL'S Fat Free Devil's Food Cookie Cakes	1 cookie	11.88
Okra, frozen, cooked	1 cup	11.79
Soup, vegetarian vegetable, canned, prepared with equal volume water	1 cup	11.78

Description	Measure	Carbs (g)
Cookies, peanut butter, prepared from recipe	1 cookie	11.78
Milk, buttermilk, fluid, cultured, lowfat	1 cup	11.74
Milk, reduced fat, fluid, 2% milkfat, with added vitamin A and vitamin D	1 cup	11.71
Milk, whole, 3.25% milkfat, with added vitamin D	1 cup	11.71
Soup, clam chowder, manhattan, canned, prepared with equal volume water	1 cup	11.64
Rutabagas, cooked	1 cup	11.63
Tortillas, ready-to-bake or -fry, corn	1 tortilla	11.61
Watermelon, raw	1 cup	11.48
Frozen novelties, ice type, pop	1 bar	11.35
Cookies, fig bars	1 cookie	11.34
Peaches, canned, juice pack	1 half	11.34
Bread, Multi-Grain, toasted	1 slice	11.31
Carrots, frozen, cooked	1 cup	11.29
Peas, edible-podded, boiled	1 cup	11.28
Soup, minestrone, canned, prepared with equal volume water	1 cup	11.23
Tangerines, (mandarin oranges), raw	1 tangerine	11.21
Broccoli, cooked	1 cup	11.20
Candies, fudge, vanilla with nuts	1 piece	11.19
Kiwifruit, green, raw	1 medium	11.14
Crackers, whole-wheat	4 crackers	11.13
Raisins, seedless	1 packet	11.09

Description	Measure	Carbs (g)
Brussels sprouts, cooked	1 cup	11.08
Cookies, molasses	1 cookie	11.07
Kohlrabi, cooked	1 cup	11.04
Vegetable juice cocktail, canned	1 cup	11.01
Pancakes, plain, dry mix, prepared	1 cake	10.98
Cucumber, with peel, raw	1 large	10.93
Cherries, sweet, raw	10 cherries	10.89
Cookies, vanilla sandwich with creme filling	1 cookie	10.82
Cocoa mix, no sugar added, powder	1/2 oz	10.79
Cocoa mix, powder, prepared with water	1 serving	10.77
Graham crackers (plain or honey)	2 squares	10.75
Collards, cooked	1 cup	10.74
Plums, canned, purple, heavy syrup	1 plum	10.69
Yogurt, plain, whole milk	8-oz	10.58
Carrots, raw	1 cup	10.54
Cheese, cottage, with fruit	1 cup	10.42
Tomato juice, canned, with salt added	1 cup	10.30
Onions, raw	1 whole	10.27
Baking chocolate, unsweetened, liquid	1 oz	10.26
Cookies, oatmeal, with raisins	1 cookie	10.26
Bread, reduced-calorie, white	1 slice	10.19

Description	Measure	Carbs (g)
Cookies, sugar, regular (includes vanilla)	1 cookie	10.19
Sauerkraut, canned, solids and liquids	1 cup	10.10
Turkey patties, breaded, battered, fried	1 patty	10.05
Bread, italian	1 slice	10.00
Grapefruit, raw, white, all areas	1/2 grapefruit	9.92
Soup, vegetable beef, canned, prepared with equal volume water	1 cup	9.91
Pineapple, canned, heavy syrup	1 slice	9.90
Oyster, cooked, breaded and fried	3 oz	9.88
Cookies, oatmeal, soft-type	1 cookie	9.86
Beans, snap, yellow, cooked	1 cup	9.85
Beans, snap, green, cooked	1 cup	9.85
Cookies, sugar, refrigerated dough, baked	1 cookie	9.84
Pears, canned, juice pack	1 half	9.83
Bread, reduced-calorie, wheat	1 slice	9.77
Shrimp, cooked, breaded and fried	3 oz	9.75
Cheese, cottage, nonfat	1 cup	9.66
Soup, chunky chicken noodle, canned	1 cup	9.60
Tomatoes, red, canned, packed in juice	1 cup	9.60
Cereals ready-to-eat, wheat, puffed	1 cup	9.55
Onions, cooked, boiled	1 medium	9.54
Scallop, cooked, breaded and fried	6 large	9.42

Description	Measure	Carbs (g)
Peaches, raw	1 peach	9.35
Cookies, chocolate chip, made with margarine	1 cookie	9.34
Bread, reduced-calorie, rye	1 slice	9.32
Soup, cream of chicken, canned, prepared with equal volume water	1 cup	9.27
Nuts, cashew nuts, dry roasted, with salt added	1 oz	9.27
Soup, chicken noodle, mix, prepared with water	1 cup	9.26
MORNINGSTAR FARMS Grillers Burger Style	1 cup	9.13
Spinach, frozen, chopped or leaf, cooked	1 cup	9.12
Peppers, sweet, red, cooked	1 cup	9.11
Peppers, sweet, green, cooked	1 cup	9.11
Grapes, red or green (Thompson seedless)	10 grapes	9.05
Peppers, sweet, red, raw	1 cup	8.98
Orange juice, raw	1 orange	8.94
Crackers, saltines (includes oyster, soda, soup)	4 crackers	8.92
Crackers, rye, wafers, plain	1 wafer	8.84
Cookies, peanut butter, regular	1 cookie	8.84
Soup, beef noodle, canned, prepared with equal volume water	1 cup	8.74
Beans, snap, yellow, frozen, cooked	1 cup	8.71
Beans, snap, green, frozen, cooked	1 cup	8.71
Cookies, oatmeal, commercially prepared	1 cookie	8.65
Eggplant, cooked	1 cup	8.64

Description	Measure	Carbs (g)
Nuts, cashew nuts, oil roasted, salt added	18 nuts	8.55
Taco shells, baked	1 medium	8.52
Baking chocolate, unsweetened, squares	1 square	8.46
Cookies, sugar, prepared from recipe	1 cookie	8.40
Cheese, cottage, lowfat, 2% milkfat	1 cup	8.27
Cabbage, cooked, boiled	1 cup	8.27
Mushrooms, white, cooked, boiled	1 cup	8.25
Fish, herring, Atlantic, pickled	3 oz	8.20
Turnip greens, frozen, cooked	1 cup	8.17
Cookies, shortbread, pecan	1 cookie	8.16
Soup, cream of mushroom, canned, prepared with equal volume water	1 cup	8.13
Nuts, pistachio nuts, dry roasted, with salt added	1 oz (47 nuts)	8.13
Carrots, canned, regular pack, drained solids	1 cup	8.09
Spinach souffle	1 cup	8.02
Snacks, popcorn, cakes	1 cake	8.01
Sugars, powdered	1 tbsp	7.98
Mushrooms, canned, drained solids	1 cup	7.94
Leeks, (bulb and lower leaf-portion), cooked	1 cup	7.92
Turnips, cooked, boiled	1 cup	7.89
Beet greens, cooked, boiled	1 cup	7.86
Chicken, thigh, meat and skin, fried, battered	1 thigh	7.81

Description	Measure	Carbs (g)
Candies, caramels	1 piece	7.78
Squash, summer, all varieties, cooked	1 cup	7.76
MORNINGSTAR FARMS Grillers Vegan	1 patty	7.74
Sunflower seeds, dry roasted, with salt	1/4 cup	7.70
Plums, raw	1 plum	7.54
Cheese, ricotta, whole milk	1 cup	7.48
Pineapple, canned, juice pack	1 slice	7.38
Crackers, standard snack-type, regular	4 crackers	7.36
Cornstarch	1 tbsp	7.36
Onions, spring or scallions (includes tops and bulb)	1 cup	7.34
Rice cakes, brown rice, plain	1 cake	7.34
Cookies, chocolate chip, regular	1 cookie	7.33
Kale, cooked, boiled	1 cup	7.32
Spinach, canned, regular pack, drained solids	1 cup	7.28
Carambola, (starfruit), raw	1 cup	7.27
Fruit butters, apple	1 tbsp	7.22
Okra, cooked, boiled	1 cup	7.22
Cookies, vanilla sandwich, creme filling	1 cookie	7.21
Nuts, mixed nuts, dry roasted, with peanuts, with salt added	1 oz	7.19
Peppers, sweet, red, raw	1 pepper	7.18
Carob flour	1 tbsp	7.11

Description	Measure	Carbs (g)
Soup, chicken noodle, canned, prepared with equal volume water	1 cup	7.11
Cheese, cottage, creamed, large or small curd	1 cup	7.10
Cookies, chocolate sandwich, creme filling	1 cookie	7.07
Sauce, hoisin, ready-to-serve	1 tbsp	7.05
Soup, chicken with rice, canned, prepared with equal volume water	1 cup	7.04
Tomatoes, red, ripe, raw, year round average	1 cup	7.00
Plums, canned, purple, juice pack	1 plum	6.97
Peppers, sweet, green, raw	1 cup	6.91
Carrots, raw	1 carrot	6.90
Nuts, coconut meat, raw	1 piece	6.85
Candies, milk chocolate coated raisins	10 pieces	6.84
Fish, catfish, channel, breaded and fried	3 oz	6.83
Sunflower seeds, dry roasted, with salt added	1 oz	6.82
Soup, onion, dry, mix, prepared with water	1 cup	6.81
Spinach, cooked, boiled	1 cup	6.75
Cauliflower, frozen, cooked, boiled	1 cup	6.75
Dandelion greens, cooked, boiled	1 cup	6.72
Syrups, pancake, reduced-calorie	1 tbsp	6.68
Sauce, barbecue	1 tbsp	6.42
Doughnuts, cake-type, plain (includes unsugared, old-fashioned)	1 hole	6.39
Cookies, chocolate chip, commercially prepared	1 cookie	6.39

Description	Measure	Carbs (g)
Mustard greens, cooked, boiled	1 cup	6.31
Popcorn, air-popped	1 cup	6.23
Doughnuts, yeast-leavened, glazed (includes honey buns)	1 hole	6.23
Mung beans, mature seeds, sprouted, raw	1 cup	6.18
Cheese, cottage, lowfat, 1% milkfat	1 cup	6.15
Nuts, almonds	24 nuts	6.14
Candies, caramels, chocolate-flavor roll	1 piece	6.14
Carambola, (starfruit), raw	1 fruit	6.12
Peanuts, dry-roasted, with salt	approx 28	6.10
Beans, snap, yellow, canned	1 cup	6.08
Cucumber, peeled, raw	1 large	6.05
Celery, cooked, boiled	1 cup	6.00
Nuts, mixed nuts, oil roasted, with peanuts	1 oz	5.97
Chicken, drumstick, meat and skin, battered	1 drumstick	5.96
Crackers, cheese, regular	10 crackers	5.94
Fish, fish portions and sticks, frozen	1 stick	5.93
Candies, hard	1 piece	5.88
Broccoli, raw	1 cup	5.84
Alcoholic beverage, beer, light	12 fl oz	5.81
Beans, snap, green, canned	1 cup	5.74
Popcorn, cheese-flavor	1 cup	5.68

Description	Measure	Carbs (g)
Melons, cantaloupe, raw	1/8 melon	5.63
Peppers, sweet, green, raw	1 pepper	5.52
Lemons, raw, without peel	1 lemon	5.41
Crackers, wheat, regular	4 crackers	5.39
Chicken, wing, meat and skin, fried, battered	1 wing	5.36
Pickle relish, sweet	1 tbsp	5.26
Mung beans, , sprouted, cooked	1 cup	5.20
Shrimp, cooked, breaded and fried	6 large	5.16
Cookies, shortbread, plain	1 cookie	5.16
Cabbage, red, raw	1 cup	5.16
NESTLE, BUTTERFINGER Bar	1 fun size bar	5.10
Salad dressing, french dressing, reduced fat	1 tbsp	5.09
Candies, SPECIAL DARK Chocolate Bar	1 miniature	5.08
Clam, mixed species, canned	3 oz	5.02
M&M's Milk Chocolate Candies	10 pieces	4.98
Beets, cooked, boiled, drained	1 beet	4.98
Cauliflower, raw	1 cup	4.97
Popcorn, oil-popped, regular flavor	1 cup	4.96
Gelatin desserts, dry mix, reduced calorie	1/2 cup	4.94
Salad dressing, russian dressing	1 tbsp	4.88
Tomatoes, red, ripe, raw, year round average	1 tomato	4.78

Description	Measure	Carbs (g)
Salad, vegetable, tossed, without dressing, with cheese and egg	1-1/2 cups	4.75
Nuts, hazelnuts or filberts	1 oz	4.73
Salad dressing, russian dressing, low calorie	1 tbsp	4.50
Beef, liver, cooked, pan-fried	3 oz	4.39
Peanuts, all types, oil-roasted, with salt	1 oz	4.33
Crackers, sandwich, with cheese filling	1 sandwich	4.32
Sauce, cheese, ready-to-serve	1/4 cup	4.30
Cabbage, savoy, raw	1 cup	4.27
Peppers, hot chili, green, raw	1 pepper	4.26
Bamboo shoots, canned, drained solids	1 cup	4.22
Sugars, granulated	1 tsp	4.20
Pumpkin and squash seeds, roasted, salted	1 oz	4.17
Alcoholic beverage, daiquiri	2 fl oz	4.16
Onions, dehydrated flakes	1 tbsp	4.16
Candies, gumdrops, starch jelly pieces	1 medium	4.15
STARBURST Fruit Chews, Original fruits	1 piece	4.13
Cabbage, raw	1 cup	4.06
Crackers, cheese, sandwich-type with peanut butter filling	1 sandwich	3.97
Peppers, hot chili, red, raw	1 pepper	3.96
Catsup	1 tbsp	3.93
Nuts, pecans	20 halves	3.93

Description	Measure	Carbs (g)
Apricots, raw	1 apricot	3.89
Nuts, walnuts, english	14 halves	3.89
Squash, summer, all varieties, raw	1 cup	3.79
Cucumber, with peel, raw	1 cup	3.78
Salad, vegetable, tossed, with chicken	1-1/2 cups	3.73
Nuts, pine nuts, dried	1 oz	3.71
Salad dressing, thousand island	1 tbsp	3.68
Nuts, macadamia nuts, dry roasted, salted	10-12 nuts	3.64
Lettuce, butterhead (includes boston and bibb types)	1 head	3.63
Celery, raw	1 cup	3.56
Cereals ready-to-eat, wheat germ, toasted	1 tbsp	3.53
Nuts, brazilnuts, dried, unblanched	6-8 nuts	3.48
Asparagus, frozen, cooked, boiled	1 cup	3.46
Peanut butter, chunk style, with salt	1 tbsp	3.45
Cookies, butter, commercially prepared	1 cookie	3.45
Gravy, mushroom, canned	1/4 cup	3.26
Lemon juice, raw	of 1 lemon	3.24
Gravy, chicken, canned, ready-to-serve	1/4 cup	3.22
Lime juice, raw	of 1 lime	3.20
Sesame butter, tahini, from roasted and toasted kernels (most common type)	1 tbsp	3.18
Sugars, brown	1 tsp	3.14

Description	Measure	Carbs (g)
Peanut butter, smooth style, with salt	1 tbsp	3.13
Cocoa, dry powder, unsweetened	1 tbsp	3.13
Bologna, beef and pork	2 slices	3.11
Leavening agents, yeast, baker's, compressed	1 cake	3.08
Gravy, turkey, canned, ready-to-serve	1/4 cup	3.04
Mollusks, clam, mixed species, raw	3 oz	3.03
Cabbage, chinese (pak-choi), cooked, boiled	1 cup	3.03
Cookies, vanilla wafers, lower fat	1 cookie	2.94
Candies, hard	1 small piece	2.94
Cabbage, chinese (pe-tsai), cooked, boiled	1 cup	2.87
Gravy, beef, canned, ready-to-serve	1/4 cup	2.80
Sauce, teriyaki, ready-to-serve	1 tbsp	2.80
Mushrooms, shiitake, dried	1 mushroom	2.71
Alcoholic beverage, wine, table, red	3.5 fl oz	2.69
Alcoholic beverage, wine, table, white	3.5 fl oz	2.68
Chicken roll, light meat	2 slices	2.64
Turkey roast, boneless, light and dark meat	3 oz	2.61
Cucumber, peeled, raw	1 cup	2.57
Cheese spread, process, American	1 oz	2.47
Asparagus, cooked, boiled, drained	4 spears	2.47
Avocados, raw, California	1 oz	2.45

Description	Measure	Carbs (g)
Salad dressing, french dressing	1 tbsp	2.43
Cheese food, process, American, vitamin D fortified	1 oz	2.43
Salad dressing, home recipe, cooked	1 tbsp	2.38
Leavening agents, baking powder	1 tsp	2.35
Mollusks, oyster, eastern, wild, raw	6 medium	2.28
Mushrooms, white, raw	1 cup	2.28
Avocados, raw, Florida	1 oz	2.22
Snacks, beef jerky, chopped and formed	1 large piece	2.18
Chicken, dark meat, meat only, fried	3 oz	2.18
Ham, regular (approximately 11% fat)	2 slices	2.17
Tofu, soft	1 piece	2.16
Broccoli, raw	1 spear	2.06
Spices, garlic powder	1 tsp	2.04
Hummus, commercial	1 tbsp	2.00
Tomatillos, raw	1 medium	1.99
Spices, cinnamon, ground	1 tsp	1.85
Leavening agents, cream of tartar	1 tsp	1.85
Lettuce, cos or romaine, raw	1 cup	1.84
Sandwich spread, pork, beef	1 tbsp	1.79
Salad dressing, italian dressing	1 tbsp	1.78
Asparagus, canned, drained solids	4 spears	1.77

Description	Measure	Carbs (g)
Soup, beef broth, bouillon, consomme, prepared with equal volume water	1 cup	1.76
Braunschweiger (a liver sausage), pork	2 slices	1.76
Beets, canned, drained solids	1 beet	1.73
Pickles, cucumber, dill or kosher dill	1 pickle	1.68
Shallots, raw	1 tbsp	1.68
Endive, raw	1 cup	1.68
Frankfurter, beef, unheated	1 frank	1.67
Spices, onion powder	1 tsp	1.66
Lettuce, iceberg (includes crisphead types)	1 cup	1.63
Lemonade, with non-nutritive sweetener, powder, prepared with water	8 fl oz	1.61
Lettuce, green leaf, raw	1 cup	1.61
Chicken, breast, meat and skin, fried, floured	1/2 breast	1.61
Catsup	1 packet	1.57
Cheese, swiss	1 oz	1.53
Hearts of palm, canned	1 piece	1.52
Strawberries, raw	1 berry	1.38
Olives, ripe, canned (small-extra large)	5 large	1.38
Tofu, firm	1/4 block	1.37
Salami, cooked, beef and pork	2 slices	1.36
Cheese, process, American, fortified with vitamin D	1 oz	1.36
Spices, pepper, black	1 tsp	1.34

Description	Measure	Carbs (g)
Spices, chili powder	1 tsp	1.29
Frankfurter, chicken	1 frank	1.23
Peppers, jalapeno, canned	1/4 cup	1.23
Cheese, cream, fat free	1 tbsp	1.19
Celery, raw	1 stalk	1.19
Spices, curry powder	1 tsp	1.16
Cheese, feta	1 oz	1.16
Spices, paprika	1 tsp	1.13
Tomatoes, sun-dried	1 piece	1.12
Spinach, raw	1 cup	1.09
Cheese, mozzarella, part skim milk	1 oz	1.09
Sauce, salsa, ready-to-serve	1 tbsp	1.08
Soup, beef broth or bouillon, powder, dry	1 packet	1.04
Tea, instant, sweetened with non-nutritive sweetener, lemon-flavored	8 fl oz	1.04
Spices, oregano, dried	1 tsp	1.03
Lime juice, canned or bottled, unsweetened	1 tbsp	1.03
Carbonated beverage, low calorie, cola or pepper-type	12 fl oz	1.03
Cheese, neufchatel	1 oz	1.02
Coffee, brewed, espresso	2 fl oz	1.00
Garlic, raw	1 clove	0.99
Seaweed, kelp, raw	2 tbsp	0.96

Description	Measure	Carbs (g)
Sesame seeds, dried (decorticated)	1 tbsp	0.94
Ham, chopped, not canned	2 slices	0.88
Spices, celery seed	1 tsp	0.83
Carrots, baby, raw	1 medium	0.82
Soy sauce made from soy and wheat (shoyu)	1 tbsp	0.79
Beef, cured, dried	1 oz	0.78
Frankfurter, beef and pork	1 frank	0.77
Salad dressing, blue or roquefort cheese	1 tbsp	0.71
Pork and beef sausage, fresh, cooked	2 links	0.70
Tomatoes, sun-dried, packed in oil	1 piece	0.70
Alfalfa seeds, sprouted, raw	1 cup	0.69
Dessert topping, powdered, 1.5 ounce prepared with 1/2 cup milk	1 tbsp	0.69
Cheese, blue	1 oz	0.66
Spices, parsley, dried	1 tbsp	0.66
Cream, fluid, half and half	1 tbsp	0.65
Dessert topping, pressurized	1 tbsp	0.64
Cream, sour, reduced fat, cultured	1 tbsp	0.64
Parsley, fresh	10 sprigs	0.63
Pork, cured, canadian-style bacon	2 slices	0.63
Cheese, mozzarella, whole milk	1 oz	0.62
Pimento, canned	1 tbsp	0.61

Description	Measure	Carbs (g)
Coffee, instant, regular	6 fl oz	0.61
Cheese, provolone	1 oz	0.61
Egg, yolk, raw, fresh	1 large	0.60
Cheese, pasteurized process, swiss	1 oz	0.60
Cheese, cream	1 tbsp	0.59
Horseradish, prepared	1 tsp	0.56
Sour dressing, non-butterfat, cultured	1 tbsp	0.56
Egg, whole, cooked, hard-boiled	1 large	0.56
Cheese, low fat, cheddar or colby	1 oz	0.54
Tea, black, brewed, prepared with water	6 fl oz	0.53
Vanilla extract	1 tsp	0.53
Salad dressing, french, home recipe	1 tbsp	0.48
Peppers, sweet, green, raw	1 ring	0.46
Cream, fluid, heavy whipping	1 tbsp	0.42
Pork, cured, ham, lean and regular, canned	3 oz	0.42
Sausage, Vienna, canned, chicken, beef, pork	1 sausage	0.42
Tea, instant, unsweetened, powder, prepared	8 fl oz	0.40
Salad dressing, home recipe, vinegar and oil	1 tbsp	0.39
Cream, whipped, cream topping, pressurized	1 tbsp	0.37
Cheese, cheddar	1 oz	0.36
Tea, herb, chamomile, brewed	6 fl oz	0.36

Description	Measure	Carbs (g)
Cream, sour, cultured	1 tbsp	0.35
Lettuce, cos or romaine, raw	1 leaf	0.33
Cheese, muenster	1 oz	0.32
Crab, blue, crab cakes	1 cake	0.29
Ham, sliced, (96% fat free, water added)	2 slices	0.28
Pork, cured, bacon, cooked	3 slices	0.27
Mustard, prepared, yellow	1 tsp	0.27
Egg, white, raw, fresh	1 large	0.24
Lettuce, iceberg (includes crisphead types)	1 medium	0.24
Salami, dry or hard, pork, beef	2 slices	0.24
Seaweed, spirulina, dried	1 tbsp	0.22
Cheese, parmesan, grated	1 tbsp	0.20
Cheese, camembert	1 wedge	0.17
Chicken, liver, all classes, cooked	1 liver	0.17
Radishes, raw	1 radish	0.15
Vinegar, cider	1 tbsp	0.14
Chives, raw	1 tbsp	0.13
Margarine, regular, 80% fat, composite	1 tbsp	0.11
Margarine-like, vegetable oil spread	1 tbsp	0.10
Sauce, ready-to-serve, pepper or hot	1 tsp	0.08
Salad dressing, mayonnaise, regular	1 tbsp	0.08
Dill weed, fresh	5 sprigs	0.07

Description	Measure	Carbs (g)
Margarine-like, vegetable oil spread, approximately 37% fat, with salt	1 tsp	0.03
Butter, salted	1 tbsp	0.01
Pork (all except liver)	3 oz	0.00
Oil, sesame, salad or cooking	1 tbsp	0.00
Beef (all except liver)	3 oz	0.00
Fish (all kinds)	3 oz	0.00
Veal (all kinds)	3 oz	0.00
Oil, peanut, salad or cooking	1 tbsp	0.00
Shellfish (all kinds except Conch)	3 oz	0.00
Oil, soybean, salad or cooking, (partially hydrogenated)	1 tbsp	0.00
Oil, canola	1 tbsp	0.00
Oil, corn, industrial and retail, all purpose salad or cooking	1 tbsp	0.00
Oil, safflower, salad or cooking, high oleic (primary safflower oil of commerce)	1 tbsp	0.00
Oil, sunflower, linoleic, (approx. 65%)	1 tbsp	0.00
Coffee, brewed from grounds, prepared with tap water	6 fl oz	0.00
Oil, olive, salad or cooking	1 tbsp	0.00
Chicken (all except liver)	1 piece	0.00
Shortening, household, soybean (partially hydrogenated), cottonseed	1 tbsp	0.00
Carbonated beverage, club soda	12 fl oz	0.00
Lard	1 tbsp	0.00
Turkey (all except liver)	3 oz	0.00
Duck (all except liver)	1/2 duck	0.00

Description	Measure	Carbs (g)

Notes

Appendix B

Sorted Alphabetically

Selected Items From

USDA National Nutrient Database for Standard Reference, Release 25

Content of Selected Foods per Common Measure,
Carbohydrate, by difference (g)

Description	Measure	Carbs (g)
Alcoholic beverage, beer, light	12 fl oz	5.81
Alcoholic beverage, beer, regular, all	12 fl oz	12.60
Alcoholic beverage, daiquiri, prepared-from-recipe	2 fl oz	4.16
Alcoholic beverage, distilled, (gin, rum, vodka, whiskey)	1.5 fl oz	0.00
Alcoholic beverage, liqueur, coffee, 53 proof	1.5 fl oz	24.34
Alcoholic beverage, pina colada, prepared-from-recipe	4.5 fl oz	31.95
Alcoholic beverage, wine, dessert, dry	3.5 fl oz	12.02
Alcoholic beverage, wine, dessert, sweet	3.5 fl oz	14.10
Alcoholic beverage, wine, table, red	3.5 fl oz	2.69
Alcoholic beverage, wine, table, white	3.5 fl oz	2.68
Alfalfa seeds, sprouted, raw	1 cup	0.69
Apple juice, canned or bottled, unsweetened	1 cup	28.02
Apples, dried, sulfured, uncooked	5 rings	21.08
Apples, raw, with skin	1 apple	19.06
Apples, raw, without skin	1 cup	14.04
Applesauce, canned, sweetened	1 cup	44.60
Applesauce, canned, unsweetened	1 cup	27.50
Apricot nectar, canned	1 cup	36.12
Apricots, canned, heavy syrup pack	1 cup	55.39
Apricots, canned, juice pack, with skin	1 cup	30.11
Apricots, dried, sulfured, uncooked	10 halves	21.92
Apricots, raw	1 apricot	3.89
Artichokes, (globe or french), cooked	1 choke	14.34
Asparagus, canned, drained solids	4 spears	1.77
Asparagus, cooked, boiled, drained	4 spears	2.47
Asparagus, frozen, cooked, boiled, drained	4 spears	1.15
Avocados, raw	1 oz	2.45
Bagels, cinnamon-raisin	4" bagel	49.13
Bagels, egg	4" bagel	47.17

Description	Measure	Carbs (g)
Bagels, plain, enriched, with calcium propionate	4" bagel	44.95
Baking chocolate, unsweetened, liquid	1 oz	10.26
Baking chocolate, unsweetened, squares	1 square	8.46
Bamboo shoots, canned, drained solids	1 cup	4.22
Bananas, raw	1 banana	26.95
Barley, pearled, cooked	1 cup	44.31
Barley, pearled, raw	1 cup	155.4
Beans, baked, canned, plain or vegetarian	1 cup	53.70
Beans, baked, canned, with franks	1 cup	39.86
Beans, baked, canned, with pork and sweet sauce	1 cup	53.36
Beans, baked, canned, with pork and tomato sauce	1 cup	47.29
Beans, black, mature seeds, cooked, boiled	1 cup	40.78
Beans, great northern, mature seeds, cooked	1 cup	37.33
Beans, kidney, red, mature seeds, canned	1 cup	37.96
Beans, kidney, red, mature seeds, cooked	1 cup	40.36
Beans, navy, mature seeds, cooked, boiled	1 cup	47.41
Beans, pinto, mature seeds, cooked, boiled	1 cup	44.84
Beans, snap, green, canned, regular pack	1 cup	5.74
Beans, snap, green, cooked, boiled, drained	1 cup	9.85
Beans, snap, green, frozen, cooked, boiled	1 cup	8.71
Beans, snap, yellow, canned, regular pack	1 cup	6.08
Beans, snap, yellow, cooked, boiled, drained	1 cup	9.85
Beans, snap, yellow, frozen, cooked, boiled	1 cup	8.71
Beans, white, mature seeds, canned	1 cup	55.54
Beef stew, canned entree	1 cup	18.21
Beef (all kinds, except liver)	3 oz	0.00
Beef, variety meats and by-products, liver, pan-fried	3 oz	4.39
Beet greens, cooked, boiled, drained	1 cup	7.86

Description	Measure	Carbs (g)
Beets, canned, drained solids	1 cup	12.26
Beets, cooked, boiled, drained	1 cup	16.93
Barley, pearled, cooked	1 cup	44.31
Barley, pearled, raw	1 cup	155.4
Beans, baked, canned, plain or vegetarian	1 cup	53.70
Beans, baked, canned, with franks	1 cup	39.86
Beans, baked, canned, with pork and sweet sauce	1 cup	53.36
Beans, baked, canned, with pork and tomato sauce	1 cup	47.29
Beans, black, mature seeds, cooked, boiled	1 cup	40.78
Beans, great northern, mature seeds, cooked	1 cup	37.33
Beans, kidney, red, mature seeds, canned	1 cup	37.96
Beans, kidney, red, mature seeds, cooked	1 cup	40.36
Beans, navy, mature seeds, cooked, boiled	1 cup	47.41
Beans, pinto, mature seeds, cooked, boiled	1 cup	44.84
Beans, snap, green, canned, regular pack	1 cup	5.74
Beans, snap, green, cooked, boiled, drained	1 cup	9.85
Beans, snap, green, frozen, cooked, boiled	1 cup	8.71
Beans, snap, yellow, canned, regular pack	1 cup	6.08
Beans, snap, yellow, cooked, boiled, drained	1 cup	9.85
Beans, snap, yellow, frozen, cooked, boiled	1 cup	8.71
Beans, white, mature seeds, canned	1 cup	55.54
Beef stew, canned entree	1 cup	18.21
Beef (all kinds, except liver)	3 oz	0.00
Beef, variety meats and by-products, liver, pan-fried	3 oz	4.39
Beet greens, cooked, boiled, drained	1 cup	7.86
Beets, canned, drained solids	1 cup	12.26
Beets, cooked, boiled, drained	1 cup	16.93
Biscuits, plain or buttermilk, prepared from recipe	2-1/2" biscuit	26.76

Description	Measure	Carbs (g)
Biscuits, plain or buttermilk, prepared from recipe	4" biscuit	45.05
Biscuits, plain or buttermilk, higher fat, baked	2-1/2" biscuit	12.59
Biscuits, plain or buttermilk, lower fat, baked	2-1/4" biscuit	11.63
Blackberries, raw	1 cup	13.84
Blueberries, frozen, sweetened	1 cup	50.49
Blueberries, raw	1 cup	21.01
Bologna, beef and pork	2 slices	3.11
Braunschweiger (a liver sausage), pork	2 slices	1.76
Bread crumbs, dry, grated, plain	1 oz	20.41
Bread crumbs, dry, grated, seasoned	1 cup	82.19
Bread stuffing, bread, dry mix, prepared	1/2 cup	21.70
Bread, banana, prepared from recipe	1 slice	32.76
Bread, cornbread, dry mix, prepared	1 piece	32.67
Bread, cracked-wheat	1 slice	12.38
Bread, egg	1/2" slice	19.12
Bread, french or vienna (includes sourdough)	1/2" slice	14.11
Bread, italian	1 slice	10.00
Bread, Multi-Grain (includes whole-grain)	1 slice	11.27
Bread, oatmeal	1 slice	13.10
Bread, pita, white, enriched	4" pita	15.60
Bread, pita, white, enriched	6-1/2" pita	33.42
Bread, pumpernickel	1 slice	15.20
Bread, raisin, enriched	1 slice	13.60
Bread, raisin, toasted, enriched	1 slice	13.66
Bread, reduced-calorie, rye	1 slice	9.32
Bread, reduced-calorie, wheat	1 slice	9.77
Bread, reduced-calorie, white	1 slice	10.19
Bread, rye	1 slice	15.46
Bread, wheat	1 slice	12.37

Description	Measure	Carbs (g)
Bread, white (includes soft bread crumbs)	1 slice	12.27
Bread, whole-wheat, commercially prepared	1 slice	11.56
Broccoli, cooked, boiled, drained, without salt	1 cup	11.20
Broccoli, flower clusters, raw	1 floweret	0.58
Brussels sprouts, cooked, boiled, drained	1 cup	11.08
Buckwheat groats, roasted, cooked	1 cup	33.50
Bulgur, cooked	1 cup	33.82
Bulgur, dry	1 cup	106.22
Butter, salted	1 tbsp	0.01
Butter, without salt	1 tbsp	0.01
Cabbage, chinese (pak-choi), cooked	1 cup	3.03
Cabbage, chinese (pe-tsai), cooked	1 cup	2.87
Cabbage, cooked, boiled, drained	1 cup	8.27
Cabbage, raw	1 cup	4.06
Cabbage, red, raw	1 cup	5.16
Cabbage, savoy, raw	1 cup	4.27
Cake, angelfood, commercially prepared	1 piece	16.18
Cake, angelfood, dry mix, prepared	1 piece	29.35
Cake, boston cream pie	1 piece	39.47
Cake, chocolate, commercially prepared with chocolate	1 piece	33.82
Cake, chocolate, prepared from recipe without frosting	1 piece	50.73
Cake, fruitcake, commercially prepared	1 piece	26.49
Cake, gingerbread, prepared from recipe	1 piece	36.41
Cake, pineapple upside-down	1 piece	58.08
Cake, pound, commercially prepared, butter	1 piece	13.66
Cake, pound, commercially prepared, fat-free	1 slice	17.08
Cake, shortcake, biscuit-type	1 cake	31.53
Cake, snack cakes, creme-filled, chocolate with frosting	1 cupcake	30.16
Cake, snack cakes, creme-filled, sponge	1 cake	27.21
Cake, snack cakes, cupcakes, chocolate, with frosting	1 cupcake	28.90

Description	Measure	Carbs (g)
Cake, sponge, commercially prepared	1 cake	18.33
Cake, sponge, prepared from recipe	1 piece	36.35
Cake, white, with coconut frosting	1 piece	70.78
Cake, white, prepared from recipe without frosting	1 piece	42.33
Cake, yellow, with chocolate frosting	1 piece	35.43
Cake, yellow, with vanilla frosting	1 piece	37.63
Candies, caramels	1 piece	7.78
Candies, caramels, chocolate-flavor roll	1 piece	6.14
Candies, carob, unsweetened	1 oz	15.96
Candies, fudge, chocolate, prepared-from-recipe	1 piece	12.99
Candies, fudge, chocolate, with nuts	1 piece	12.91
Candies, fudge, vanilla with nuts	1 piece	11.19
Candies, fudge, vanilla, prepared-from-recipe	1 piece	13.14
Candies, gumdrops, starch jelly pieces	10 worms	73.19
Candies, gumdrops, starch jelly pieces	1 medium	4.15
Candies, gumdrops, starch jelly pieces	10 bears	21.76
Candies, hard	1 small piece	2.94
Candies, hard	1 piece	5.88
Candies, jellybeans	10 large	26.52
Candies, KIT KAT Wafer Bar	1 bar	27.13
Candies, M&M's Milk Chocolate	10 pieces	4.98
Candies, M&M's Peanut Chocolate	10 pieces	12.10
Candies, MILKY WAY Bar	1 fun size bar	12.81
Candies, MILKY WAY Bar	1 bar	43.41
Candies, SNICKERS Bar	1 bar	35.06
Candies, STARBURST Fruit Chews	1 piece	4.13
Candies, marshmallows	1 cup	40.65
Candies, milk chocolate	1 bar	26.14

Description	Measure	Carbs (g)
Candies, milk chocolate coated peanuts	10 pieces	19.88
Candies, milk chocolate coated raisins	10 pieces	6.84
Candies, milk chocolate, with almonds	1 bar	21.89
Candies, MR. GOODBAR Chocolate Bar	1 bar	26.63
Candies, NESTLE, BUTTERFINGER Bar	1 fun size bar	5.10
Candies, NESTLE, CRUNCH Bar and Dessert Topping	1 bar	29.48
Candies, REESE'S Peanut Butter Cups	2	24.91
Candies, semisweet chocolate	1 cup	107.35
Candies, SPECIAL DARK Chocolate Bar	1 miniature	5.08
Candies, white chocolate	1 cup	100.71
Carambola, (starfruit), raw	1 cup	7.27
Carambola, (starfruit), raw	1 fruit	6.12
Carbonated beverage, club soda	12 fl oz	0.00
Carbonated beverage, cola, contains caffeine	12 fl oz	35.37
Carbonated beverage, ginger ale	12 fl oz	32.10
Carbonated beverage, grape soda	12 fl oz	41.66
Carbonated beverage, low calorie, cola or pepper-type	12 fl oz	1.03
Carbonated beverage, low calorie, not cola or pepper	12 fl oz	0.00
Carbonated beverage, orange	12 fl oz	45.76
Carbonated beverage, pepper-type	12 fl oz	38.27
Carbonated beverage, root beer	12 fl oz	39.22
Carbonated beverage, SPRITE, lemon-lime	12 fl oz	37.32
Carob flour	1 tbsp	7.11
Carrot juice, canned	1 cup	21.90
Carrots, baby, raw	1 medium	0.82
Carrots, canned, regular pack, drained solids	1 cup	8.09
Carrots, cooked, boiled, drained, without salt	1 cup	12.82
Carrots, frozen, cooked, boiled, drained	1 cup	11.29

Description	Measure	Carbs (g)
Carrots, raw	1 cup	10.54
Carrots, raw	1 carrot	6.90
Catsup	1 tbsp	3.93
Catsup	1 packet	1.57
Cauliflower, cooked, boiled, drained	1 cup	5.10
Cauliflower, raw	1 cup	4.97
Celery, cooked, boiled, drained, without salt	1 cup	6.00
Celery, raw	1 cup	3.56
Cereals, Corn CHEX	1 cup	25.47
Cereals, APPLE CINNAMON CHEERIOS	3/4 cup	24.39
Cereals, BASIC 4	1 cup	43.56
Cereals, BERRY BERRY KIX	3/4 cup	25.14
Cereals, CHEERIOS	1 cup	21.97
Cereals, CINNAMON TOAST CRUNCH	3/4 cup	23.92
Cereals, COCOA PUFFS	1 cup	25.11
Cereals, GOLDEN GRAHAMS	3/4 cup	25.53
Cereals, HONEY NUT CHEERIOS	1 cup	23.97
Cereals, Honey Nut CHEX	3/4 cup	26.25
Cereals, HONEY NUT CLUSTERS	1 cup	46.86
Cereals, KIX	1-1/3 cup	24.85
Cereals, LUCKY CHARMS	1 cup	24.27
Cereals, RAISIN NUT BRAN	1 cup	44.28
Cereals, REESE'S PUFFS	3/4 cup	22.68
Cereals, Rice CHEX	1-1/4 cup	26.20
Cereals, TOTAL Raisin Bran	1 cup	42.24
Cereals, TRIX	1 cup	25.68
Cereals, Wheat CHEX	1 cup	24.66
Cereals, WHEATIES	1 cup	24.99
Cereals, Whole Grain TOTAL	3/4 cup	22.41

Description	Measure	Carbs (g)
Cereals, KELLOGG'S ALL-BRAN COMPLETE Wheat Flakes	3/4 cup	22.91
Cereals, KELLOGG'S ALL-BRAN Original	1/2 cup	22.27
Cereals, KELLOGG'S APPLE JACKS	1 cup	26.46
Cereals, KELLOGG'S COCOA KRISPIES	3/4 cup	26.68
Cereals, KELLOGG'S Corn Flakes	1 cup	23.55
Cereals, KELLOGG'S CORN POPS	1 cup	28.02
Cereals, KELLOGG'S CRISPIX	1 cup	24.85
Cereals, KELLOGG'S FROOT LOOPS	1 cup	26.01
Cereals, KELLOGG'S FROSTED FLAKES	3/4 cup	27.65
Cereals, KELLOGG'S FROSTED MINI-WHEATS	1 cup	46.39
Cereals, KELLOGG'S HONEY SMACKS	3/4 cup	23.90
Cereals, KELLOGG'S PRODUCT 19	1 cup	24.90
Cereals, KELLOGG'S RAISIN BRAN	1 cup	47.15
Cereals, KELLOGG'S RICE KRISPIES	1-1/4 cup	28.07
Cereals, KELLOGG'S RICE KRISPIES TREATS	3/4 cup	25.41
Cereals, KELLOGG'S SPECIAL K	1 cup	22.63
Cereals, KELLOGG'S FROSTED MINI-WHEATS, Big Bite	1 cup	43.04
Cereals, QUAKER, CAP'N CRUNCH	3/4 cup	23.09
Cereals, QUAKER, CAP'N CRUNCH CRUNCHBERRIES	3/4 cup	22.33
Cereals, QUAKER, CAP'N CRUNCH'S PEANUT BUTTER CRUNCH	3/4 cup	21.24
Cereals, QUAKER, Low Fat 100% Natural Granola with Raisins	1/2 cup	40.29
Cereals, QUAKER, QUAKER 100% Natural Granola with Oats, Wheat, Honey, and Raisins	1/2 cup	38.08
Cereals, QUAKER OAT CINNAMON LIFE	3/4 cup	25.33
Cereals, QUAKER OAT LIFE, plain	3/4 cup	24.88

Description	Measure	Carbs (g)
Cereals, rice, puffed, fortified	1 cup	12.57
Cereals, wheat germ, toasted, plain	1 tbsp	3.53
Cereals, wheat, puffed, fortified	1 cup	9.55
Cereals, wheat, shredded, plain, sugar free	2 biscuits	36.23
Cereals, corn grits, white, regular and quick, enriched	1 cup	35.72
Cereals, corn grits, yellow, regular and quick, enriched	1 cup	33.54
Cereals, CREAM OF WHEAT, mix'n eat	1 packet	21.44
Cereals, CREAM OF WHEAT, regular (10 minute)	1 cup	26.41
Cereals, farina, enriched, assorted brands including CREAM	1 cup	26.10
Cereals, Malt-o-Meal, plain, prepared with water	1serving	23.37
Cereals, oats, instant, fortified, plain,prepared with water	1 packet	20.66
Cereals, oats, regular and quick, unenriched, cooked	1 cup	28.08
Cereals, QUAKER, corn grits, instant, plain, prepared (microwaved or boiling water added), without salt	1 packet	21.85
Cereals, WHEATENA, cooked with water	1 cup	28.67
Cheese food, pasteurized process, American	1 oz	2.43
Cheese sauce, prepared from recipe	1 cup	13.32
Cheese spread, pasteurized process, American	1 oz	2.47
Cheese, blue	1 oz	0.66
Cheese, camembert	1 wedge	0.17
Cheese, cheddar	1 oz	0.36
Cheese, cottage, creamed, large or small curd	1 cup	7.10
Cheese, cottage, creamed, with fruit	1 cup	10.42
Cheese, cottage, lowfat, 1% milkfat	1 cup	6.15

Description	Measure	Carbs (g)
Cheese, cottage, lowfat, 2% milkfat	1 cup	8.27
Cheese, cottage, nonfat, uncreamed, dry, large or small curd	1 cup	9.66
Cheese, cream	1 tbsp	0.59
Cheese, cream, fat free	1 tbsp	1.19
Cheese, feta	1 oz	1.16
Cheese, low fat, cheddar or colby	1 oz	0.54
Cheese, mozzarella, part skim milk, low moisture	1 oz	1.09
Cheese, mozzarella, whole milk	1 oz	0.62
Cheese, muenster	1 oz	0.32
Cheese, neufchatel	1 oz	1.02
Cheese, parmesan, grated	1 tbsp	0.20
Cheese, pasteurized process, American	1 oz	1.36
Cheese, pasteurized process, Swiss	1 oz	0.60
Cheese, provolone	1 oz	0.61
Cheese, ricotta, part skim milk	1 cup	12.64
Cheese, ricotta, whole milk	1 cup	7.48
Cheese, Swiss	1 oz	1.53
Cheesecake commercially prepared	1 piece	20.40
Cherries, sour, red, canned	1 cup	21.81
Cherries, sweet, raw	10 cherries	10.89
Chicken pot pie, frozen entree, prepared	1 small pie	41.21
Chicken roll, light meat	2 slices	2.64
Chicken, broilers or fryers, breast, meat only, roasted	1/2 breast	0.00
Chicken, broilers or fryers, dark meat, drumstick	1 drumstick	0.00
Chicken, broilers or fryers, dark meat, meat only, fried, battered	3 oz	2.18
Chicken, broilers or fryers, drumstick, meat and skin, fried, battered	1 drumstick	5.96

Description	Measure	Carbs (g)
Chicken, broilers or fryers, drumstick, meat and skin	1 drumstick	0.80
Chicken, broilers or fryers, giblets, simmered	1 cup	0.00
Chicken, broilers or fryers, light meat, meat only, fried	3 oz	0.35
Chicken, broilers or fryers, thigh, meat and skin, fried, battered	1 thigh	7.81
Chicken, broilers or fryers, thigh, meat only, roasted	1 thigh	0.00
Chicken, broilers or fryers, wing, meat and skin, fried, battered	1 wing	5.36
Chicken, canned, meat only, with broth	5 oz	0.00
Chicken, liver, all classes, cooked, simmered	1 liver	0.17
Chicken, stewing, meat only, cooked, stewed	1 cup	0.00
Chickpeas (garbanzo beans, bengal gram), mature seeds, canned	1 cup	32.38
Chickpeas (garbanzo beans, bengal gram), mature seeds, cooked, boiled, without salt	1 cup	44.97
Chili con carne with beans, canned entree	1 cup	29.08
Chives, raw	1 tbsp	0.13
Chocolate syrup	1 tbsp	12.21
Chocolate-flavor beverage mix for milk, powder	2-3 large tsp	19.63
Chocolate-flavor beverage mix, powder, prepared with whole milk	1 cup	31.68
Cocoa mix, no sugar added, powder	1/2 oz envelope	10.79
Cocoa mix, powder	3 tsp	23.74
Cocoa mix, powder, prepared with water	1 serving	23.77
Cocoa mix, with aspartame, powder, prepared with water	1 serving	10.77
Cocoa, dry powder, unsweetened	1 tbsp	3.13
Coffee, brewed from grounds, prepared with tap water	6 fl oz	0.00
Coffee, brewed, espresso	2 fl oz	1.00

Description	Measure	Carbs (g)
Coffee, instant, regular, prepared with water	6 fl oz	0.61
Coffeecake, cinnamon with crumb topping, commercially prepared, enriched	1 piece	29.42
Coleslaw, home-prepared	1 cup	14.89
Collards, cooked, boiled, drained	1 cup	10.74
Collards, frozen, chopped, cooked	1 cup	12.07
Cookies, brownies, commercially prepared	1 brownie	35.78
Cookies, brownies, dry mix, special dietary	1 brownie	15.69
Cookies, butter, commercially prepared	1 cookie	3.45
Cookies, chocolate chip, commercially prepared, higher fat, enriched	1 cookie	6.39
Cookies, chocolate chip, commercially prepared, regular, lower fat	1 cookie	7.33
Cookies, chocolate chip, prepared from recipe, made with margarine	1 cookie	9.34
Cookies, chocolate chip, refrigerated dough, baked	1 cookie	17.73
Cookies, chocolate sandwich, with creme filling, regular	1 cookie	7.07
Cookies, fig bars	1 cookie	11.34
Cookies, graham crackers, plain or honey	2 squares	10.75
Cookies, graham crackers, plain or honey	1 cup	64.51
Cookies, molasses	1 cookie, medium	11.07
Cookies, molasses	1 cookie, large	23.62
Cookies, oatmeal, commercially prepared, fat-free	1 cookie	8.65
Cookies, oatmeal, commercially prepared, regular	1 cookie	17.18
Cookies, oatmeal, commercially prepared, soft-type	1 cookie	9.86
Cookies, oatmeal, prepared from recipe, with raisins	1 cookie	10.26
Cookies, peanut butter, prepared from recipe	1 cookie	11.78

Description	Measure	Carbs (g)
Cookies, shortbread, commercially prepared, pecan	1 cookie	8.16
Cookies, shortbread, commercially prepared, plain	1 cookie	5.16
Cookies, sugar, commercially prepared, regular	1 cookie	10.19
Cookies, sugar, prepared from recipe, with margarine	1 cookie	8.40
Cookies, sugar, refrigerated dough, baked	1 cookie	9.84
Cookies, vanilla sandwich with creme filling	1 cookie	10.82
Cookies, vanilla wafers, lower fat	1 cookie	2.94
Corn, sweet, white, cooked, boiled	1 ear	16.72
Corn, sweet, yellow, canned, cream style	1 cup	46.41
Corn, sweet, yellow, canned, vacuum pack	1 cup	40.82
Corn, sweet, yellow, cooked, boiled	1 ear	16.15
Corn, sweet, yellow, frozen, kernels cut off cob, drained	1 cup	31.65
Corn, sweet, yellow, frozen, kernels on cob, cooked	1 ear	14.07
Cornmeal, degermed, enriched, yellow	1 cup	109.64
Cornmeal, self-rising, degermed, enriched, yellow	1 cup	103.21
Cornmeal, whole-grain, yellow	1 cup	93.81
Cornstarch	1 tbsp	7.36
Couscous, cooked	1 cup	36.46
Couscous, dry	1 cup	133.95
Cowpeas (blackeyes), immature seeds, cooked	1 cup	33.53
Cowpeas, common (blackeyes, crowder, southern)	1 cup	32.71
Cowpeas, common (blackeyes, crowder, southern), mature seeds, cooked, boiled	1 cup	35.71
Crackers, cheese, regular	10	5.94

Description	Measure	Carbs (g)
Crackers, cheese, sandwich-type with peanut butter filling	1 sandwich	3.97
Crackers, matzo, plain	1 matzo	23.73
Crackers, melba toast, plain	4 pieces	15.32
Crackers, rye, wafers, plain	1 wafer	8.84
Crackers, saltines (includes oyster, soda, soup)	4 crackers	8.92
Crackers, standard snack-type, regular	4 crackers	7.36
Crackers, standard snack-type, sandwich, with cheese filling	1 sandwich	4.32
Crackers, wheat, regular	4 crackers	5.39
Crackers, whole-wheat	4 crackers	11.13
Cranberry juice cocktail, bottled	8 fl oz	34.21
Cranberry sauce, canned, sweetened	1 slice	22.17
Cream substitute, liquid, with hydrogenated vegetable oil	1 tbsp	1.71
Cream substitute, powdered	1 tsp	1.10
Cream, fluid, half and half	1 tbsp	0.65
Cream, fluid, heavy whipping	1 tbsp	0.42
Cream, fluid, light (coffee cream or table cream)	1 tbsp	0.55
Cream, fluid, light whipping	1 tbsp	0.44
Cream, sour, cultured	1 tbsp	0.35
Cream, sour, reduced fat, cultured	1 tbsp	0.64
Cream, whipped, cream topping, pressurized	1 tbsp	0.37
Croissants, butter	1	26.11
Croutons, seasoned	1 cup	25.40
Crustaceans, crab, alaska king, cooked	3 oz	0.00
Crustaceans, crab, alaska king, imitation, made from surimi	3 oz	12.75
Crustaceans, crab, blue, canned	1 cup	0.00

Description	Measure	Carbs (g)
Crustaceans, crab, blue, cooked, moist heat	3 oz	0.00
Crustaceans, crab, blue, crab cakes	1 cake	0.29
Crustaceans, lobster, northern, cooked	3 oz	0.00
Crustaceans, shrimp, mixed species, canned	3 oz	0.00
Crustaceans, shrimp, mixed species, breaded and fried	6 large	5.16
Crustaceans, shrimp, mixed species, breaded and fried	3 oz	9.75
Cucumber, peeled, raw	1 large	6.05
Cucumber, peeled, raw	1 cup	2.57
Cucumber, with peel, raw	1 cup	3.78
Cucumber, with peel, raw	1 large	10.93
Dandelion greens, boiled, drained	1 cup	6.72
Danish pastry, cheese	1 danish	26.41
Danish pastry, fruit, enriched (includes apple, cinnamon, raisin, lemon, raspberry, strawberry)	1 danish	33.94
Dates, deglet noor	5 dates	31.14
Dates, deglet noor	1 cup	133.55
Dessert topping, powdered, 1.5 ounce prepared with 1/2 cup milk	1 tbsp	0.69
Dessert topping, pressurized	1 tbsp	0.64
Dessert topping, semi solid, frozen	1 tbsp	0.92
Dill weed, fresh	5 sprigs	0.07
Doughnuts, cake-type, plain (includes unsugared)	1 medium	21.45
Doughnuts, yeast-leavened, glazed, enriched	1 medium	28.76
Duck, domesticated, meat only, roasted	1/2 duck	0.00
Eclairs, custard-filled with chocolate glaze, from recipe	1 eclair	24.20
Egg, white, raw, fresh	1 large	0.24
Egg, whole, cooked, fried	1 large	0.38

Description	Measure	Carbs (g)
Egg, whole, cooked, hard-boiled	1 large	0.56
Egg, whole, cooked, poached	1 large	0.36
Egg, whole, cooked, scrambled	1 large	0.98
Egg, whole, raw, fresh	1 medium	0.32
Egg, whole, raw, fresh	1 large	0.36
Egg, whole, raw, fresh	1 extra large	0.42
Egg, yolk, raw, fresh	1 large	0.60
Eggnog	1 cup	20.45
Eggplant, cooked, boiled, drained	1 cup	8.64
Endive, raw	1 cup	1.68
English muffins, plain, toasted, enriched, with calcium propionate (includes sourdough)	1 muffin	27.38
Entrees, fish fillet, battered or breaded, and fried	1 fillet	15.44
Fast Food, Pizza Chain, 14" pizza, pepperoni topping, regular crust	1 slice	33.90
Fast Foods, biscuit, with egg and sausage	1 biscuit	37.89
Fast foods, burrito, with beans and beef	1 burrito	22.55
Fast foods, burrito, with beans and cheese	1 burrito	29.04
Fast foods, cheeseburger, double, regular patty and bun, plain	1 sandwich	47.82
Fast foods, cheeseburger; double, regular patty, with condiments and vegetables	1 sandwich	35.19
Fast foods, cheeseburger; double, regular patty; plain	1 sandwich	32.24
Fast foods, cheeseburger; single, large patty; with condiments and bacon	1 sandwich	36.84
Fast foods, cheeseburger; single, large patty; with condiments and vegetables	1 sandwich	36.81
Fast foods, cheeseburger; single, regular patty, with condiments	1 sandwich	28.77
Fast foods, cheeseburger; single, regular patty; plain	1 sandwich	30.49
Fast foods, chicken fillet sandwich, plain	1 sandwich	38.69

Description	Measure	Carbs (g)
Fast foods, chicken, breaded and fried	6 pieces	15.83
Fast foods, chili con carne	1 cup	21.94
Fast foods, chimichanga, with beef	1 chimi	42.80
Fast foods, clams, breaded and fried	3/4 cup	38.81
Fast foods, coleslaw	3/4 cup	14.74
Fast foods, croissant, with egg, cheese	1 croissant	23.65
Fast foods, danish pastry, cheese	1 pastry	28.69
Fast foods, danish pastry, fruit	1 pastry	45.06
Fast foods, enchilada, with cheese	1 enchilada	28.54
Fast foods, english muffin, with egg, cheese, and canadian bacon	1 muffin	29.69
Fast foods, fish sandwich, with tartar sauce and cheese	1 sandwich	48.29
Fast foods, french toast sticks	5 sticks	58.11
Fast foods, french toast with butter	2 slices	36.05
Fast foods, frijoles with cheese	1 cup	28.71
Fast foods, hamburger; double, large patty; with condiments and vegetables	1 sandwich	40.27
Fast foods, hamburger; double, regular patty; with condiments	1 sandwich	38.74
Fast foods, hamburger; single, large patty; with condiments and vegetables	1 sandwich	40.00
Fast foods, hamburger; single, regular patty; with condiments	1 sandwich	31.34
Fast foods, hotdog, plain	1 sandwich	18.03
Fast foods, hotdog, with chili	1 sandwich	31.29
Fast foods, hotdog, with corn flour coating (corndog)	1 corn dog	55.79
Fast foods, hush puppies	5 pieces	31.36
Fast foods, nachos, with cheese	6-8 nachos	36.33
Fast foods, onion rings, breaded and fried	8-9 rings	36.17
Fast foods, pancakes with butter and syrup	2 pancakes	90.90

Description	Measure	Carbs (g)
Fast foods, potato, french fried in vegetable oil	1 small	35.22
Fast foods, potato, french fried in vegetable oil	1 large	70.03
Fast foods, potato, french fried in vegetable oil	1 medium	55.53
Fast foods, potato, mashed	1/3 cup	11.72
Fast foods, potatoes, hashed brown	1/2 cup	23.18
Fast foods, roast beef sandwich, plain	1 sandwich	33.44
Fast foods, salad, vegetable, tossed, without dressing, with cheese and egg	1-1/2 cups	4.75
Fast foods, salad, vegetable, tossed, without dressing, with chicken	1-1/2 cups	3.73
Fast foods, shrimp, breaded and fried	6-8 shrimp	45.90
Fast foods, submarine sandwich, with cold cuts	1 sandwich, 6"	51.05
Fast foods, submarine sandwich, with roast beef	1 sandwich, 6"	44.30
Fast foods, submarine sandwich, with tuna salad	1 sandwich, 6"	55.37
Fast foods, sundae, hot fudge	1 sundae	47.67
Fast foods, taco salad	1-1/2 cups	23.58
Fast foods, taco with beef, cheese and lettuce, hard shell	1 large	52.21
Fast foods, taco with beef, cheese and lettuce, hard shell	1 small	33.94
Fast foods, tostada, with beans, beef, and cheese	1 tostada	29.66
Fast foods, vanilla, light, soft-serve ice cream, with cone	1 cone	27.15
Figs, dried, uncooked	2 figs	24.27
Fish, catfish, channel, cooked, breaded and fried	3 oz	6.83
Fish, fish portions and sticks, frozen, preheated	1 portion	12.07
Fish, fish portions and sticks, frozen, preheated	1 stick	5.93
Fish (all kinds, not breaded or battered)	1 fillet	0.00

Description	Measure	Carbs (g)
Fish, herring, Atlantic, pickled	3 oz	8.20
Frankfurter, beef and pork	1 frank	0.77
Frankfurter, beef, unheated	1 frank	1.67
Frankfurter, chicken	1 frank	1.23
French toast, frozen, ready-to-heat	1 slice	18.94
French toast, prepared from recipe, made with low fat (2%) milk	1 slice	16.25
Frostings, chocolate, creamy, ready-to-eat	1/12 package	24.02
Frostings, vanilla, creamy, ready-to-eat	1/12 package	25.80
Frozen novelties, fruit and juice bars	1 bar	15.55
Frozen novelties, ice type, italian, restaurant-prepared	1/2 cup	15.66
Frozen novelties, ice type, pop	1 bar	11.35
Frozen yogurts, chocolate, soft-serve	1/2 cup	17.93
Frozen yogurts, vanilla, soft-serve	1/2 cup	17.42
Fruit butters, apple	1 tbsp	7.22
Fruit cocktail, (peach and pineapple and pear and grape and cherry), canned, syrup	1 cup	46.90
Fruit cocktail, (peach and pineapple and pear and grape and cherry), canned	1 cup	28.11
Fruit punch drink, with added nutrients	8 fl oz	29.69
Frybread, made with lard (Navajo)	10-1/2" bread	77.22
Frybread, made with lard (Navajo)	5" bread	43.43
Garlic, raw	1 clove	0.99
Gelatin desserts, dry mix, prepared with water	1/2 cup	19.16
Gelatin desserts, dry mix, reduced calorie, with aspartame, prepared with water	1/2 cup	4.94
Grape drink, canned	8 fl oz	39.38
Grape juice cocktail, frozen concentrate, diluted with 3 volume water	1 cup	31.88
Grape juice cocktail, frozen concentrate, undiluted, with added ascorbic acid	6-fl-oz can	95.84

Description	Measure	Carbs (g)
Grape juice, canned or bottled, unsweetened, without added ascorbic acid	1 cup	37.37
Grapefruit juice, pink, raw	1 cup	22.72
Grapefruit juice, white, canned, sweetened	1 cup	27.83
Grapefruit juice, white, canned, unsweetened	1 cup	22.13
Grapefruit juice, white, frozen concentrate, unsweetened, diluted with 3 volume water	1 cup	24.03
Grapefruit juice, white, frozen concentrate, unsweetened, undiluted	6-fl-oz can	71.54
Grapefruit juice, white, raw	1 cup	22.72
Grapefruit, raw, pink and red, all areas	1/2 grapefruit	13.11
Grapefruit, raw, white, all areas	1/2 grapefruit	9.92
Grapefruit, sections, canned, light syrup pack, solids and liquids	1 cup	39.22
Grapes, red or green (European type, such as Thompson seedless), raw	1 cup	28.96
Grapes, red or green (European type, such as Thompson seedless), raw	10 grapes	9.05
Gravy, beef, canned, ready-to-serve	1/4 cup	2.80
Gravy, chicken, canned, ready-to-serve	1/4 cup	3.22
Gravy, mushroom, canned	1/4 cup	3.26
Gravy, turkey, canned, ready-to-serve	1/4 cup	3.04
Ham, chopped, not canned	2 slices	0.88
Ham, sliced, prepackaged (96% fat free, water added)	2 slices	0.28
Ham, sliced, regular (approximately 11% fat)	2 slices	2.17
Hearts of palm, canned	1 piece	1.52
Honey	1 tbsp	17.30
Horseradish, prepared	1 tsp	0.56
Hummus, commercial	1 tbsp	2.00
Ice creams, chocolate	1/2 cup	18.61
Ice creams, french vanilla, soft-serve	1/2 cup	19.09

Description	Measure	Carbs (g)
Ice creams, vanilla	1/2 cup	15.58
Ice creams, vanilla, light	1/2 cup	19.44
Ice creams, vanilla, rich	1/2 cup	16.49
Jams and preserves	1 tbsp	13.77
Jellies	1 tbsp	13.29
Jerusalem-artichokes, raw	1 cup	26.16
Kale, cooked, boiled, drained, without salt	1 cup	7.32
Kale, frozen, cooked, boiled, drained, without salt	1 cup	6.80
KELLOGG'S, EGGO, Waffles, Homestyle, Low Fat	1 waffle	15.72
Kiwifruit, green, raw	1 medium	11.14
Kohlrabi, cooked, boiled, drained, without salt	1 cup	11.04
Lamb (all kinds except liver)	3 oz	0.00
Lard	1 tbsp	0.00
Leavening agents, baking powder, double-acting	1 tsp	1.27
Leavening agents, baking soda	1 tsp	0.00
Leavening agents, cream of tartar	1 tsp	1.85
Leavening agents, yeast, baker's, active dry	1 pkg	2.89
Leeks, (bulb and lower leaf-portion), cooked, boiled, drained, without salt	1 cup	7.92
Lemon juice, canned or bottled	1 cup	15.81
Lemon juice, canned or bottled	1 tbsp	0.98
Lemon juice, raw	juice of 1 lemon	3.24
Lemonade, frozen concentrate, white, prepared with water	8 fl oz	25.84
Lemonade, low calorie, with non-nutritive sweetener, powder, prepared with water	8 fl oz	1.61
Lemonade-flavor drink, powder, prepared with water	8 fl oz	18.35
Lemons, raw, without peel	1 lemon	5.41
Lentils, mature seeds, cooked, boiled	1 cup	39.86

Description	Measure	Carbs (g)
Lettuce, butterhead (includes boston and bibb types), raw	1 medium leaf	0.17
Lettuce, butterhead (includes boston and bibb types), raw	1 head	3.63
Lettuce, cos or romaine, raw	1 leaf	0.33
Lettuce, cos or romaine, raw	1 cup	1.84
Lettuce, green leaf, raw	1 cup	1.61
Lettuce, green leaf, raw	1 leaf	0.29
Lettuce, iceberg (includes crisphead types), raw	1 medium	0.24
Lettuce, iceberg (includes crisphead types), raw	1 cup	1.63
Lettuce, iceberg (includes crisphead types), raw	1 head	16.01
Lima beans, immature seeds, frozen, baby, cooked, boiled, drained, without salt	1 cup	35.01
Lima beans, immature seeds, frozen, fordhook, cooked, boiled, drained	1 cup	32.84
Lima beans, large, mature seeds, canned	1 cup	35.93
Lima beans, large, mature seeds, cooked, boiled, without salt	1 cup	39.25
Lime juice, canned or bottled, unsweetened	1 cup	16.46
Lime juice, canned or bottled, unsweetened	1 tbsp	1.03
Lime juice, raw	1 lime	3.20
Macaroni and Cheese, canned entree	1 cup	29.03
Macaroni and cheese, frozen entree	1 package	48.90
Macaroni, cooked, enriched	1 cup	43.20
Malted drink mix, chocolate, with added nutrients, powder	3 tsp	17.77
Malted drink mix, chocolate, with added nutrients, powder, prepared with whole milk	1 cup	29.65
Malted drink mix, natural, with added nutrients, powder	4-5 heaping tsp	17.55
Malted drink mix, natural, with added nutrients, powder prepared with whole milk	1 cup	28.28

Description	Measure	Carbs (g)
Mangos, raw	1 mango	31.01
Mangos, raw	1 cup	24.72
Margarine, regular, 80% fat, composite, stick, with salt	1 tbsp	0.10
Margarine, regular, 80% fat, composite, tub, with salt	1 tbsp	0.11
Margarine-like, margarine-butter blend, soybean oil and butter	1 tbsp	0.11
Margarine-like, vegetable oil spread, 60% fat, stick, with salt	1 tsp	0.03
Margarine-like, vegetable oil spread, 60% fat, stick, with salt	1 tbsp	0.10
Margarine-like, vegetable oil spread, 60% fat, tub, with salt	1 tsp	0.04
Margarine-like, vegetable oil spread, unspecified oils, approximately 37% fat	1 tsp	0.03
Melons, cantaloupe, raw	1/8 melon	5.63
Melons, cantaloupe, raw	1 cup	13.06
Melons, honeydew, raw	1 cup	15.45
Melons, honeydew, raw	1/8 melon	14.54
Milk shakes, thick chocolate	10.6 fl oz	63.45
Milk shakes, thick vanilla	11 fl oz	55.56
Milk, buttermilk, dried	1 tbsp	3.19
Milk, buttermilk, fluid, cultured, lowfat	1 cup	11.74
Milk, canned, condensed, sweetened	1 cup	166.46
Milk, canned, evaporated, nonfat, with added vitamin A and vitamin D	1 cup	29.06
Milk, canned, evaporated, with added vitamin D and without added vitamin A	1 cup	25.30
Milk, chocolate, fluid, commercial, lowfat, with added vitamin A and vitamin D	1 cup	31.50
Milk, chocolate, fluid, commercial, reduced fat, with added vitamin A and D	1 cup	30.33
Milk, chocolate, fluid, commercial, whole, with added vitamin A and vitamin D	1 cup	25.85
Milk, dry, nonfat, instant, with added vitamin A and vitamin D	1/3 cup	12.00

Description	Measure	Carbs (g)
Milk, lowfat, fluid, 1% milkfat, with added vitamin A and vitamin D	1 cup	12.18
Milk, nonfat, fluid, with added vitamin A and vitamin D (fat free or skim)	1 cup	12.15
Milk, reduced fat, fluid, 2% milkfat, with added vitamin A and vitamin D	1 cup	11.71
Milk, whole, 3.25% milkfat, with added vitamin D	1 cup	11.71
Miso	1 cup	18.20
Mollusks, clam, mixed species, canned	3 oz	5.02
Mollusks, clam, mixed species, raw	3 oz	3.03
Mollusks, oyster, eastern, cooked, breaded and fried	3 oz	9.88
Mollusks, oyster, eastern, wild, raw	6 medium	2.28
Mollusks, scallop, mixed species, cooked, breaded and fried	6 large	9.42
MORNINGSTAR FARMS Grillers Burger Style Recipe Crumbles, frozen, unprepared	1 cup	9.13
MORNINGSTAR FARMS Grillers Vegan, frozen, unprepared	1 patty	7.74
Muffins, blueberry, commercially prepared (Includes mini- muffins)	1 muffin	30.77
Muffins, blueberry, prepared from recipe, made with low fat (2%) milk	1 muffin	23.20
Muffins, corn, commercially prepared	1 muffin	29.01
Muffins, corn, dry mix, prepared	1 muffin	24.55
Muffins, oat bran	1 muffin	27.53
Muffins, wheat bran, toaster-type with raisins, toasted	1 muffin	18.87
Mung beans, mature seeds, sprouted, cooked, boiled, drained, without salt	1 cup	5.20
Mung beans, mature seeds, sprouted, raw	1 cup	6.18
Mushrooms, canned, drained solids	1 cup	7.94
Mushrooms, shiitake, cooked, without salt	1 cup	20.87
Mushrooms, shiitake, dried	1 mushroom	2.71
Mushrooms, white, cooked, boiled, drained, without salt	1 cup	8.25

Description	Measure	Carbs (g)
Mushrooms, white, raw	1 cup	2.28
Mustard greens, cooked, boiled	1 cup	6.31
Mustard, prepared, yellow	1 tsp or 1 packet	0.27
NABISCO, NABISCO SNACKWELL'S Fat Free Devil's Food	1 cookie	11.88
Nectarines, raw	1	14.35
Noodles, chinese, chow mein	1 cup	30.16
Noodles, egg, cooked, enriched	1 cup	40.26
Noodles, egg, spinach, cooked, enriched	1 cup	38.80
Nuts, almonds	24 nuts	6.14
Nuts, brazilnuts, dried, unblanched	6-8 nuts	3.48
Nuts, cashew nuts, dry roasted, with salt added	1 oz	9.27
Nuts, cashew nuts, oil roasted, with salt added	18 nuts	8.55
Nuts, chestnuts, european, roasted	1 cup	75.73
Nuts, coconut meat, dried (desiccated), sweetened, shredded	1 cup	44.33
Nuts, coconut meat, raw	1 piece	6.85
Nuts, hazelnuts or filberts	1 oz	4.73
Nuts, macadamia nuts, dry roasted, with salt added	10-12 nuts	3.64
Nuts, mixed nuts, dry roasted, with peanuts, with salt added	1 oz	7.19
Nuts, mixed nuts, oil roasted, with peanuts, with salt added	1 oz	5.97
Nuts, pecans	20 halves	3.93
Nuts, pine nuts, dried	1 oz	3.71
Nuts, pine nuts, dried	1 tbsp	1.12
Nuts, pistachio nuts, dry roasted, with salt added	47 nuts	8.13
Nuts, walnuts, english	14 halves	3.89
Oat bran, cooked	1 cup	25.05
Oat bran, raw	1 cup	62.25

Description	Measure	Carbs (g)
Oil, canola	1 tbsp	0.00
Oil, corn, industrial and retail, all purpose salad or cooking	1 tbsp	0.00
Oil, olive, salad or cooking	1 tbsp	0.00
Oil, peanut, salad or cooking	1 tbsp	0.00
Oil, safflower, salad or cooking, high oleic (primary safflower oil of commerce)	1 tbsp	0.00
Oil, sesame, salad or cooking	1 tbsp	0.00
Oil, soybean, salad or cooking, (partially hydrogenated)	1 tbsp	0.00
Oil, sunflower, linoleic, (approx. 65%)	1 tbsp	0.00
Okra, cooked, boiled, drained, without salt	1 cup	7.22
Okra, frozen, cooked, boiled, drained	1 cup	11.79
Olives, ripe, canned (small-extra large)	5 large	1.38
Onion rings, breaded, par fried, frozen, prepared, heated in oven	10 rings	22.90
Onions, cooked, boiled, drained, without salt	1 medium	9.54
Onions, cooked, boiled, drained, without salt	1 cup	21.32
Onions, dehydrated flakes	1 tbsp	4.16
Onions, raw	1 cup	14.94
Onions, raw	1 whole	10.27
Onions, raw	1 slice	1.31
Onions, spring or scallions (includes tops and bulb), raw	1 whole	1.10
Onions, spring or scallions (includes tops and bulb), raw	1 cup	7.34
Orange juice, canned, unsweetened	1 cup	27.41
Orange juice, chilled, includes from concentrate	1 cup	28.73
Orange juice, frozen concentrate, unsweetened, diluted with 3 volume water	1 cup	26.84
Orange juice, frozen concentrate, unsweetened, undiluted	6-fl-oz can	81.30
Orange juice, raw	1 cup	25.79

144

Description	Measure	Carbs (g)
Orange juice, raw	1 orange	8.94
Oranges, raw, all commercial varieties	1 orange	15.39
Oranges, raw, all commercial varieties	1 cup	21.15
Pancakes plain, frozen, ready-to-heat (includes buttermilk)	1 pancake	13.59
Pancakes, plain, dry mix, complete, prepared	1 pancake	13.95
Pancakes, plain, dry mix, incomplete, prepared	1 pancake	10.98
Papayas, raw	1 cup	15.15
Papayas, raw	1 papaya	32.89
Parsley, fresh	10 sprigs	0.63
Parsnips, cooked, boiled, drained	1 cup	26.54
Pasta with meatballs in tomato sauce	1 cup	28.00
Peaches, canned, heavy syrup pack	1 cup	52.24
Peaches, canned, heavy syrup pack	1 half	19.54
Peaches, canned, juice pack	1 cup	28.69
Peaches, canned, juice pack	1 half	11.34
Peaches, dried, sulfured, uncooked	3 halves	23.92
Peaches, frozen, sliced, sweetened	1 cup	59.95
Peaches, raw	1 peach	9.35
Peaches, raw	1 cup	16.22
Peanut butter, chunk style, with salt	1 tbsp	3.45
Peanut butter, smooth style, with salt	1 tbsp	3.13
Peanuts, all types, dry-roasted, with salt	approx 28	6.10
Peanuts, all types, oil-roasted, with salt	1 oz	4.33
Pears, asian, raw	1 pear	29.29
Pears, asian, raw	1 pear	12.99
Pears, canned, heavy syrup pack	1 half	14.57
Pears, canned, heavy syrup pack	1 cup	50.99

Description	Measure	Carbs (g)
Pears, canned, juice pack, solids and liquids	1 cup	32.09
Pears, canned, juice pack	1 half	9.83
Pears, raw	1 pear	25.28
Peas, edible-podded, boiled, drained	1 cup	11.28
Peas, edible-podded, frozen, cooked	1 cup	14.43
Peas, green (includes baby and lesuer types), canned, drained solids	1 cup	19.31
Peas, green, frozen, cooked, boiled	1 cup	22.82
Peas, split, mature seeds, cooked	1 cup	41.36
Peppers, hot chili, green, raw	1 pepper	4.26
Peppers, hot chili, red, raw	1 pepper	3.96
Peppers, jalapeno, canned	1/4 cup	1.23
Peppers, sweet, green, cooked, boiled	1 cup	9.11
Peppers, sweet, green, raw	1 ring	0.46
Peppers, sweet, green, raw	1 pepper	5.52
Peppers, sweet, green, raw	1 cup	6.91
Peppers, sweet, red, cooked, boiled	1 cup	9.11
Peppers, sweet, red, raw	1 pepper	7.18
Peppers, sweet, red, raw	1 cup	8.98
Pickle relish, sweet	1 tbsp	5.26
Pickles, cucumber, dill or kosher dill	1 pickle	1.68
Pie crust, cookie-type, prepared from recipe, graham cracker, baked	1 pie shell	155.83
Pie crust, standard-type, frozen, ready-to-bake, enriched, baked	1 pie shell	70.86
Pie crust, standard-type, prepared from recipe, baked	1 pie shell	85.50
Pie fillings, apple, canned	1/8 of 21-oz can	19.31
Pie fillings, canned, cherry	1/8 of 21-oz can	20.72
Pie, apple, commercially prepared, enriched flour	1 piece	39.78

Description	Measure	Carbs (g)
Pie, apple, prepared from recipe	1 piece	57.51
Pie, blueberry, commercially prepared	1 piece	40.83
Pie, blueberry, prepared from recipe	1 piece	49.25
Pie, cherry, commercially prepared	1 piece	46.57
Pie, cherry, prepared from recipe	1 piece	69.30
Pie, chocolate creme, commercially prepared	1 piece	37.97
Pie, coconut custard, commercially prepared	1 piece	31.41
Pie, fried pies, cherry	1 pie	54.53
Pie, fried pies, fruit	1 pie	54.53
Pie, lemon meringue, commercially prepared	1 piece	53.34
Pie, lemon meringue, prepared from recipe	1 piece	49.66
Pie, pecan, commercially prepared	1 piece	67.36
Pie, pecan, prepared from recipe	1 piece	63.68
Pie, pumpkin, commercially prepared	1 piece	37.96
Pie, pumpkin, prepared from recipe	1 piece	40.92
Pimento, canned	1 tbsp	0.61
Pineapple and grapefruit juice drink	8 fl oz	29.00
Pineapple and orange juice drink, canned	8 fl oz	29.50
Pineapple juice, canned, unsweetened	1 cup	32.18
Pineapple, canned, heavy syrup pack	1 slice	9.90
Pineapple, canned, heavy syrup pack	1 cup	51.31
Pineapple, canned, juice pack	1 cup	39.09
Pineapple, canned, juice pack	1 slice	7.38
Pineapple, raw, all varieties	1 cup	20.34
Pizza, cheese topping, regular crust	1 serving	18.28
Pizza, meat and vegetable topping	1 serving	19.86
Plantains, cooked	1 cup	47.97
Plantains, raw	1 medium	57.08

Description	Measure	Carbs (g)
Plums, canned, purple, heavy syrup pack	1 cup	59.96
Plums, canned, purple, heavy syrup pack	1 plum	10.69
Plums, canned, purple, juice pack, solids	1 plum	6.97
Plums, canned, purple, juice pack, solids	1 cup	38.18
Plums, dried (prunes), stewed	1 cup	69.64
Plums, dried (prunes), uncooked	5 prunes	26.83
Plums, raw	1 plum	7.54
Pork and beef sausage, fresh, cooked	2 links	0.70
Pork sausage, fresh, cooked	2 links	0.00
Pork sausage, fresh, cooked	1 patty	0.00
Pork, cured, bacon, cooked, broiled, pan-fried or roasted	3 medium slices	0.27
Pork, cured, canadian-style bacon, grilled	2 slices	0.63
Pork, cured, ham, extra lean and regular, canned, roasted	3 oz	0.42
Pork (all kinds except liver)	3 oz	0.00
Potato pancakes	1 pancake	21.14
Potato puffs, frozen, oven-heated	10 puffs	21.92
Potato salad, home-prepared	1 cup	27.93
Potato, baked, flesh and skin, without salt	1 potato	42.72
Potatoes, au gratin, dry mix, prepared with water, whole milk and butter	1 cup	31.46
Potatoes, au gratin, home-prepared from recipe using butter	1 cup	27.61
Potatoes, baked, flesh, without salt	1 potato	33.62
Potatoes, baked, skin, without salt	1 skin	26.71
Potatoes, boiled, cooked in skin	1 potato	27.38
Potatoes, boiled, cooked without skin	1 cup	31.22
Potatoes, boiled, cooked without skin	1 potato	27.01
Potatoes, french fried, all types, salt added in processing, frozen, home-prepared, oven heated	10 strips	13.87

Description	Measure	Carbs (g)
Potatoes, hashed brown, frozen, plain, prepared	1 patty	8.15
Potatoes, hashed brown, home-prepared	1 cup	54.77
Potatoes, mashed, dehydrated, prepared from flakes without milk, whole milk and butter added	1 cup	22.83
Potatoes, mashed, home-prepared, whole milk added	1 cup	36.90
Potatoes, mashed, home-prepared, whole milk and margarine added	1 cup	35.57
Potatoes, scalloped, dry mix, prepared with water, whole milk and butter	1 cup	31.29
Potatoes, scalloped, home-prepared with butter	1 cup	26.41
Poultry food products, ground turkey, cooked	1 patty	0.00
Prune juice, canned	1 cup	44.67
Puddings, chocolate, dry mix, instant, prepared with 2% milk	1/2 cup	27.77
Puddings, chocolate, dry mix, regular, prepared with 2% milk	1/2 cup	28.06
Puddings, chocolate, ready-to-eat	4 oz	26.00
Puddings, rice, ready-to-eat	4 oz	22.00
Puddings, tapioca, ready-to-eat	4 oz	24.51
Puddings, vanilla, dry mix, regular, prepared with 2% milk	1/2 cup	25.94
Puddings, vanilla, ready-to-eat	4 oz	25.54
Pumpkin, canned, without salt	1 cup	19.82
Pumpkin, cooked, boiled, drained	1 cup	12.01
Radishes, raw	1 radish	0.15
Raisins, seedless	1 cup	114.81
Raisins, seedless	1 packet	11.09
Raspberries, frozen, red, sweetened	1 cup	65.40
Raspberries, raw	1 cup	14.69
Refried beans, canned, traditional style (includes USDA commodity)	1 cup	38.46
Rhubarb, frozen, cooked, with sugar	1 cup	74.88

Description	Measure	Carbs (g)
Rice drink, unsweetened, with added calcium, vitamins A and D	8 fl oz	22.01
Rice, brown, long-grain, cooked	1 cup	44.77
Rice, white, long-grain, parboiled, enriched, cooked	1 cup	45.59
Rice, white, long-grain, parboiled, enriched, dry	1 cup	149.65
Rice, white, long-grain, precooked or instant, enriched, prepared	1 cup	41.42
Rice, white, long-grain, regular, cooked	1 cup	44.51
Rice, white, long-grain, regular, raw	1 cup	147.91
Rolls, dinner, plain, commercially prepared (includes brown-and- serve)	1 roll	14.57
Rolls, hamburger or hotdog, plain	1 roll	21.56
Rolls, hard (includes kaiser)	1 roll	30.04
Rutabagas, cooked, boiled, drained	1 cup	11.63
Salad dressing, blue or roquefort cheese dressing, commercial, regular	1 tbsp	0.71
Salad dressing, french dressing, commercial, regular	1 tbsp	2.43
Salad dressing, french dressing, reduced fat	1 tbsp	5.09
Salad dressing, french, home recipe	1 tbsp	0.48
Salad dressing, home recipe, cooked	1 tbsp	2.38
Salad dressing, home recipe, vinegar and oil	1 tbsp	0.39
Salad dressing, italian dressing, commercial, reduced fat	1 tbsp	1.50
Salad dressing, italian dressing, commercial, regular	1 tbsp	1.78
Salad dressing, mayonnaise, regular	1 tbsp	0.08
Salad dressing, russian dressing	1 tbsp	4.88
Salad dressing, russian dressing, low calorie	1 tbsp	4.50
Salad dressing, thousand island dressing, reduced fat	1 tbsp	3.68

Description	Measure	Carbs (g)
Salad dressing, thousand island, commercial, regular	1 tbsp	2.28
Salami, cooked, beef and pork	2 slices	1.36
Salami, dry or hard, pork, beef	2 slices	0.24
Salt, table	1 tsp	0.00
Sandwich spread, pork, beef	1 tbsp	1.79
Sauce, barbecue	1 tbsp	6.42
Sauce, cheese, ready-to-serve	1/4 cup	4.30
Sauce, hoisin, ready-to-serve	1 tbsp	7.05
Sauce, homemade, white, medium	1 cup	22.93
Sauce, pasta, spaghetti/marinara	1 cup	18.83
Sauce, ready-to-serve, pepper or hot	1 tsp	0.08
Sauce, salsa, ready-to-serve	1 tbsp	1.08
Sauce, teriyaki, ready-to-serve	1 tbsp	2.80
Sauerkraut, canned, solids and liquids	1 cup	10.10
Sausage, Vienna, canned, chicken, beef, pork	1 sausage	0.42
Seaweed, kelp, raw	2 tbsp	0.96
Seaweed, spirulina, dried	1 tbsp	0.22
Seeds, pumpkin and squash seed kernels, roasted, with salt added	1 oz	4.17
Seeds, sesame butter, tahini, from roasted and toasted kernels (most common type)	1 tbsp	3.18
Seeds, sesame seed kernels, dried (decorticated)	1 tbsp	0.94
Seeds, sunflower seed kernels, dry roasted, with salt added	1/4 cup	7.70
Seeds, sunflower seed kernels, dry roasted, with salt added	1 oz	6.82
Shake, fast food, chocolate	16 fl oz	68.27
Shake, fast food, vanilla	16 fl oz	65.23
Shallots, raw	1 tbsp	1.68
Sherbet, orange	1/2 cup	22.50

Description	Measure	Carbs (g)
Shortening, household (partially hydrogenated)	1 tbsp	0.00
Snack, potato chips, made from dried potatoes, plain	1 oz	14.75
Snacks, beef jerky, chopped and formed	1 piece	2.18
Snacks, corn-based, extruded, chips, barbecue-flavor	1 oz	15.93
Snacks, corn-based, extruded, chips, plain	1 oz	17.86
Snacks, corn-based, extruded, puffs or twists, cheese-flavor	1 oz	15.03
Snacks, fruit leather, pieces	1 oz	23.48
Snacks, fruit leather, rolls	1 large	18.02
Snacks, GENERAL MILLS, CHEX MIX, traditional flavor	1 oz	21.20
Snacks, granola bars, hard, plain	1 bar	18.26
Snacks, granola bars, soft, coated, milk chocolate coating, peanut butter	1 bar	15.14
Snacks, granola bars, soft, uncoated, chocolate chip	1 bar	19.90
Snacks, granola bars, soft, uncoated, raisin	1 bar	18.82
Snacks, KELLOGG, KELLOGG'S RICE KRISPIES TREATS Squares	1 bar	17.71
Snacks, KELLOGG'S, NUTRI-GRAIN Cereal Bars, fruit	1 bar	25.73
Snacks, oriental mix, rice-based	1 oz	14.63
Snacks, popcorn, air-popped	1 cup	6.23
Snacks, popcorn, cakes	1 cake	8.01
Snacks, popcorn, caramel-coated, with peanuts	1 cup	33.89
Snacks, popcorn, caramel-coated, without peanuts	1 cup	27.84
Snacks, popcorn, cheese-flavor	1 cup	5.68
Snacks, popcorn, oil-popped, microwave, regular flavor	1 cup	4.96
Snacks, pork skins, plain	1 oz	0.00
Snacks, potato chips, barbecue-flavor	1 oz	14.97

Description	Measure	Carbs (g)
Snacks, potato chips, made from dried potatoes, reduced fat	1 oz	18.40
Snacks, potato chips, made from dried potatoes, sour-cream and onion-flavor	1 oz	14.54
Snacks, potato chips, plain, salted	1 oz	14.40
Snacks, potato chips, plain, unsalted	1 oz	15.00
Snacks, potato chips, reduced fat	1 oz	18.97
Snacks, potato chips, sour-cream-and-onion-flavor	1 oz	14.60
Snacks, pretzels, hard, plain, salted	10 pretzels	47.86
Snacks, rice cakes, brown rice, plain	1 cake	7.34
Snacks, tortilla chips, nacho cheese	1 oz	17.50
Snacks, tortilla chips, nacho-flavor, reduced fat	1 oz	20.30
Snacks, tortilla chips, plain, white corn	1 oz	18.59
Snacks, trail mix, regular, with chocolate chips, salted nuts and seeds	1 cup	65.55
Snacks, trail mix, tropical	1 cup	91.84
Soup, bean with ham, canned, chunky, ready-to-serve	1 cup	27.12
Soup, bean with pork, canned, prepared with equal volume water	1 cup	21.02
Soup, beef broth or bouillon, powder, dry	1 packet	1.04
Soup, beef broth, bouillon, consomme, prepared with equal volume water	1 cup	1.76
Soup, beef noodle, canned, prepared with equal volume water	1 cup	8.74
Soup, chicken noodle, canned, prepared with equal volume water	1 cup	7.11
Soup, chicken noodle, dry, mix, prepared with water	1 cup	9.26
Soup, chicken vegetable, chunky, canned, ready-to-serve	1 cup	18.89
Soup, chicken vegetable, chunky, reduced fat, reduced sodium, ready-to-serve, single	1 serving	14.99
Soup, chicken with rice, canned, prepared with equal volume water	1 cup	7.04
Soup, chunky chicken noodle, canned, ready-to-serve	1 cup	9.60

Description	Measure	Carbs (g)
Soup, chunky vegetable, canned, ready-to-serve	1 cup	19.01
Soup, clam chowder, manhattan, canned, prepared with equal volume water	1 cup	11.64
Soup, clam chowder, new england, canned, prepared with equal volume low	1 cup	18.50
Soup, clam chowder, new england, canned, ready-to-serve	1 cup	21.03
Soup, cream of chicken, canned, prepared with equal volume milk	1 cup	14.98
Soup, cream of chicken, canned, prepared with equal volume water	1 cup	9.27
Soup, cream of mushroom, canned, prepared with equal volume low fat (2%) milk	1 cup	14.28
Soup, cream of mushroom, canned, prepared with equal volume water	1 cup	8.13
Soup, minestrone, canned, prepared with equal volume water	1 cup	11.23
Soup, minestrone, canned, reduced sodium, ready-to-serve	1 cup	21.69
Soup, onion, dry, mix	1 packet	25.38
Soup, onion, dry, mix, prepared with water	1 cup	6.81
Soup, pea, green, canned, prepared with equal volume water	1 cup	24.70
Soup, stock, fish, home-prepared	1 cup	0.00
Soup, tomato, canned, prepared with equal volume low fat (2%) milk	1 cup	22.20
Soup, tomato, canned, prepared with equal volume water, commercial	1 cup	16.03
Soup, vegetable beef, canned, prepared with equal volume water	1 cup	9.91
Soup, vegetarian vegetable, canned, prepared with equal volume water	1 cup	11.78
Sour dressing, non-butterfat, cultured, filled cream-type	1 tbsp	0.56
Soy sauce made from soy and wheat (shoyu)	1 tbsp	0.79
Soybeans, green, cooked, boiled, drained	1 cup	19.89
Soybeans, mature cooked, boiled	1 cup	17.08
Soymilk, original and vanilla, unfortified	1 cup	15.39

Description	Measure	Carbs (g)
Spaghetti with meat sauce, frozen entree	1 package	43.13
Spaghetti, cooked, enriched	1 cup	43.20
Spaghetti, whole-wheat, cooked	1 cup	37.16
Spices, celery seed	1 tsp	0.83
Spices, chili powder	1 tsp	1.29
Spices, cinnamon, ground	1 tsp	1.85
Spices, curry powder	1 tsp	1.16
Spices, garlic powder	1 tsp	2.04
Spices, onion powder	1 tsp	1.66
Spices, oregano, dried	1 tsp	1.03
Spices, paprika	1 tsp	1.13
Spices, parsley, dried	1 tbsp	0.66
Spices, pepper, black	1 tsp	1.34
Spinach souffle	1 cup	8.02
Spinach, canned, regular pack	1 cup	7.28
Spinach, cooked, boiled, drained	1 cup	6.75
Spinach, frozen, chopped or leaf, cooked	1 cup	9.12
Spinach, raw	1 cup	1.09
Spinach, raw	1 leaf	0.36
Squash, summer, all varieties, cooked	1 cup	7.76
Squash, summer, all varieties, raw	1 cup	3.79
Squash, winter, all varieties, cooked, baked	1 cup	18.14
Squash, winter, butternut, frozen, cooked	1 cup	24.12
Strawberries, frozen, sweetened, sliced	1 cup	66.10
Strawberries, raw	1 berry	0.92
Strawberries, raw	1 cup	12.75
Strawberries, raw	1 berry	1.38
Sugars, brown	1 tsp	3.14
Sugars, granulated	1 tsp	4.20

Description	Measure	Carbs (g)
Sugars, powdered	1 tbsp	7.98
Sweet potato, canned, syrup pack	1 cup	49.71
Sweet potato, canned, vacuum pack	1 cup	53.86
Sweet potato, cooked, baked in skin	1 potato	30.24
Sweet potato, cooked, boiled, without skin	1 potato	27.64
Sweet potato, cooked, candied, home-prepared	1 piece	33.73
Sweet rolls, cinnamon, commercially prepared with raisins	1 roll	30.54
Sweet rolls, cinnamon, refrigerated dough with frosting, baked	1 roll	16.83
Syrups, chocolate, fudge-type	1 tbsp	11.95
Syrups, corn, light	1 tbsp	15.36
Syrups, maple	1 tbsp	13.41
Syrups, table blends, pancake	1 tbsp	12.29
Syrups, table blends, pancake, reduced-calorie	1 tbsp	6.68
Taco shells, baked	1 medium	8.52
Tangerine juice, canned, sweetened	1 cup	29.88
Tangerines, (mandarin oranges), canned, light syrup pack	1 cup	40.80
Tangerines, (mandarin oranges), raw	1 tangerine	11.21
Tapioca, pearl, dry	1 cup	134.81
Tea, black, brewed, prepared with tap water	6 fl oz	0.53
Tea, herb, chamomile, brewed	6 fl oz	0.36
Tea, herb, other than chamomile, brewed	6 fl oz	0.36
Tea, instant, sweetened with sugar, lemon-flavored, without added ascorbic acid, powder, prepared	8 fl oz	22.30
Tea, instant, sweetened with sweetened with non-nutritive sweetener, lemon-flavored, prepared	8 fl oz	1.04
Tea, instant, unsweetened, powder, prepared	8 fl oz	0.40
Toaster pastries, brown-sugar-cinnamon	1 pastry	34.05

Description	Measure	Carbs (g)
Toaster pastries, fruit (includes apple, blueberry, cherry, strawberry)	1 pastry	36.00
Toaster Pastries, KELLOGG, KELLOGG'S POP TARTS, Frosted chocolate fudge	1 pastry	36.61
Tofu, firm, prepared with calcium sulfate and magnesium chloride (nigari)	1/4 block	1.37
Tofu, soft, prepared with calcium sulfate and magnesium chloride (nigari)	1 piece	2.16
Tomatillos, raw	1 medium	1.99
Tomato juice, canned, with salt added	1 cup	10.30
Tomato products, canned, paste	1 cup	49.54
Tomato products, canned, puree	1 cup	22.45
Tomato products, canned, sauce	1 cup	13.18
Tomatoes, red, ripe, canned, packed in tomato juice	1 cup	9.60
Tomatoes, red, ripe, canned, stewed	1 cup	15.78
Tomatoes, red, ripe, raw, year round average	1 cup	7.00
Tomatoes, red, ripe, raw, year round average	1 slice	0.78
Tomatoes, red, ripe, raw, year round average	1 cherry tomato	0.66
Tomatoes, red, ripe, raw, year round average	1 tomato	4.78
Tomatoes, sun-dried	1 piece	1.12
Tomatoes, sun-dried, packed in oil, drained	1 piece	0.70
Tortillas, ready-to-bake or -fry, corn	1 tortilla	11.61
Tortillas, ready-to-bake or -fry, flour, refrigerated	1 tortilla	16.39
Tostada with guacamole	1 tostada	16.01
Turkey from whole, enhanced, light meat, meat only, cooked, roasted	1 serving (3 oz)	0.00
Turkey patties, breaded, battered, fried	1 patty	10.05
Turkey roast, boneless, frozen, seasoned, light and dark meat, roasted	3 oz	2.61
Turkey (all kinds except liver)	3 oz	0.00
Turnip greens, cooked, boiled, drained	1 cup	6.28

Description	Measure	Carbs (g)
Turnip greens, frozen, cooked, boiled	1 cup	8.17
Turnips, cooked, boiled, drained, without salt	1 cup	7.89
Vanilla extract	1 tsp	0.53
Veal (all kinds except liver)	3 oz	0.00
Vegetable juice cocktail, canned	1 cup	11.01
Vegetables, mixed, canned, drained solids	1 cup	15.09
Vegetables, mixed, frozen, cooked, boiled	1 cup	23.82
Vinegar, cider	1 tbsp	0.14
Waffles, plain, frozen, ready -to-heat, toasted	1 waffle	16.27
Waffles, plain, prepared from recipe	1 waffle	24.68
Water, tap, municipal	8 fl oz	0.00
Waterchestnuts, chinese, canned	1 cup	17.22
Watermelon, raw	1 cup	11.48
Watermelon, raw	1 wedge	21.59
Wheat flour, white, all-purpose, enriched, bleached	1 cup	95.39
Wheat flour, white, all-purpose, self-rising, enriched	1 cup	92.78
Wheat flour, white, bread, enriched	1 cup	99.37
Wheat flour, white, cake, enriched	1 cup	106.90
Wheat flour, whole-grain	1 cup	86.36
Wild rice, cooked	1 cup	35.00
Yogurt, fruit, low fat, 10 grams protein per 8 ounce	8-oz container	43.24
Yogurt, plain, low fat, 12 grams protein per 8 ounce	8-oz container	15.98
Yogurt, plain, skim milk, 13 grams protein per 8 ounce	8-oz container	17.43
Yogurt, plain, whole milk, 8 grams protein per 8 ounce	8-oz container	10.58

About the Author

Daryl Wein is a full-time practicing Physician Assistant in central California. He trained at U. C. Davis School of Medicine, graduating in 1999. He is a self-described "re-tread," having worked previously for twenty years as a Medical Technologist/Clinical Laboratory Scientist specializing in microbiology, hematology, clinical chemistry and immunohematology.

He resides with his wife, Jann, in Modesto, California and cares for patients in several area clinics.

He is also a licensed commercial pilot and flight instructor. His other interests include photography, music performance, water sports and amateur radio.